MW00609388

THE
AUTOIMMUNE
CURE

ALSO BY SARA SZAL GOTTFRIED, MD

Women, Food, and Hormones
The Hormone Reset Diet
Younger
Brain Body Diet
The Hormone Cure

THE
AUTOIMMUNE
CURE

Healing the Trauma and Other Triggers
That Have Turned Your Body Against You

SARA SZAL GOTTFRIED, MD

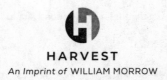

HARVEST
An Imprint of WILLIAM MORROW

FIRST EDITION

Designed by Angie Boutin

Library of Congress Cataloging-in-Publication Data has been applied for.

ISBN 978-0-06-326520-2

24 25 26 27 28 LBC 5 4 3 2 1

*To my daughters, I love you and I am working
to be the cleanest mirror for you*

CONTENTS

Introduction

Radha, whose name is Sanskrit for "devotion," is a forty-seven-year-old nutritionist and mother of two. She had suffered for years with chronic illness: irritable bowel syndrome (IBS), chronic fatigue syndrome, and fibromyalgia, which involves widespread muscle pain and discomfort, accompanied by fatigue, sleep disruptions, and poor memory and mood. Years before, she'd had a hysterectomy and partial ovary removal to alleviate chronic pelvic pain from endometriosis, fibroids, and adenomyosis. After these surgeries, she was struggling with perimenopausal symptoms, metabolic syndrome (including prediabetes and abnormal lipids), fatty liver, and high levels of inflammation and was overweight.[1]

When Radha came to see me, she was desperate for help and answers. She was frustrated that she'd suffered for so long without any true relief. Not only did she still have uncomfortable symptoms of fatigue and pain, but she didn't have any answers as to *why* she struggled with these chronic illnesses. Any previous treatment she had didn't fix the underlying issue—or it led to other, new health problems. It was like a crazy-making game of medical Whac-A-Mole with no hope in sight. She was tired of it.

As I reviewed Radha's chart and history, something jumped out at me—a pattern began to emerge. As a personalized medicine doctor, I take a deep dive into my patients' story, and there was something interesting that I'd noticed about my patients who struggled with potential autoimmune issues, like Radha. In her case, the potential autoimmune conditions were IBS and fibromyalgia.

What is autoimmunity? It's when your body's immune system—a protective system that's designed to attack invaders to keep you healthy—attacks normal, healthy tissues in the body. In other words, your body attacks itself.

The more I worked with patients who had autoimmune issues—and battled my own—the more clearly I could see a powerful, underlying connection: *trauma* was often a potential trigger for autoimmune conditions. If I went back far enough in the patient's history, more often than not I would find some form of trauma.

This hunch of mine bears out in the statistics and research. For instance, trauma has a known association with a greater risk of fibromyalgia. More than 71 percent of people with fibromyalgia meet criteria for post-traumatic stress disorder (PTSD).[2] Approximately 84 percent of fibromyalgia patients suffered one or more traumatic events prior to the onset of pain. They report traumatic events throughout their lives, including childhood and adolescence, such as emotional abuse and neglect, sexual abuse, and physical abuse. While fibromyalgia is not a classic autoimmune disease, it is nevertheless a case of the body attacking itself.

Radha had left an abusive marriage a decade prior to our first session. Interestingly, Radha's chronic conditions—the IBS, chronic fatigue, and fibromyalgia—had almost disappeared after her divorce and thanks in part to the daily spiritual practices she developed afterward: mantra, chanting, sound healing, humming, toning, restorative yoga, moving meditation with walking her labyrinth, and affirmative art.

When I began working with Radha, even though she had resolved some of the ways that her body attacked her own tissues, she still had metabolic, immune, and hormonal drift in the wrong direction. Our goal was to address the stress-related dysregulation in her physiology and cool her inflammation so that her body was less likely to develop autoimmunity. At five foot four inches and 163 pounds, she had a body mass index of 28, with significant visceral fat in her abdomen perhaps serving as a protective shield from her trauma, though also driving more inflammation.

Fast-forward three years later. Her weight is healthy at 127 pounds with a BMI of 22, her fatty liver and prediabetes are gone, and her inflammation is vastly improved, as are her lipids. She is mostly free of pain, and there is no sign of self-attack of her tissues, even after the tragic death of her beloved father one year ago. Radha is now much happier in her life and work. She has more energy to keep up with her teenaged daughters and is often mistaken for a sister rather than a mother. She looks ten years younger than when I first met her.

While Radha is not entirely free from pain, I will let her describe her experience in her own words:

"Toxic stress from past experiences became biologically embedded in my anatomy and physiology, where I was swimming in a soup of inflammation and dysregulation. This altered my ability to respond to and rebound from stressors in a healthy way. Most days I am pain-free. If I allow stress to dysregulate and derail my thoughts and choices, my fibromyalgia and fatigue will peek through the curtains as though to say, are you welcoming us back? And occasionally I surrender to the symptoms because the stressor is overwhelming, like my father's recent passing. But most days I say no and redirect my thoughts and choices moving back to pain-free, energetic existence."

Inside the body, trauma can behave like a home intruder, trespassing into your body's own physiology to wreak havoc and rob you of energy, protection, and agency. Depending on your vulnerabilities, trauma exposure may show up as heart disease, high blood sugar, depression, or another condition, like autoimmunity. While you may think you're fine, that the trauma or toxic stress you've experienced isn't a big deal, the body may not agree. Time and again, I see people who disregard their trauma, yet their body tells a different story, one of physiological dysregulation that may persist and even cause disease until the underlying forces are addressed. It was true for Radha, and it was true for me.

Who Am I?

I practice personalized medicine and serve as the director of precision medicine at the Marcus Institute of Integrative Health in Villanova, Pennsylvania, which is part of Thomas Jefferson University.[3] Precision medicine is medical care that targets optimal benefit for a particular patient or group of patients by using genetic, molecular, and biomarker profiling. Precision medicine allows for greater personalization of prevention and treatment. It may sound complex, but at its simplest, I serve people with autoimmune disease by testing genes, blood, nutrition levels, gut, stool, and hormones so we can figure out where the gaps are and how to fill them to create and achieve a mutual goal, such as peak performance, career longevity, and better relationships. I use the terms "personalized" and "precision medicine" interchangeably at times. Over the course of my career, I have practiced conventional, integrative, and functional medicine. Fundamentally, all paths lead to the same goal: you at your best, however you define that to be.

In my work, I like to offer myself as an illustration to help people learn how to be one's own case study, known as an "n-of-1" experiment (with *n* being the study's sample size—in this case, one). When I share my story, you can see what such an experiment looks like, how to conceive of it, and how to perform it—for example, how to set a body baseline as a reference point for detecting which actions lead to improvement in whatever health outcome you seek, whether it's to reduce your struggle with stress, energy, sleep, blood sugar, or autoantibodies, and take actions appropriately. For this reason, you'll read parts of my story throughout this book as a healing path that you can join. Stories become more interesting when the case faces a major health challenge, and I've struggled with my share, ranging from high antinuclear antibodies (an attack against the nucleus of my cells) to adenomyosis (an attack against the muscular wall of the uterus, leading to thickening, pain, and heavy bleeding), and from disordered eating to toxic stress.

Like Radha, I have had a life of great joy, but also tragedy. I grew up with childhood trauma and had my share of toxic stress as an adult. If we use the same adverse childhood experiences (ACE) questionnaire, Radha and I have an identical ACE score of six. (Curious about your own ACE score? See page 48 for the questionnaire used by the Institute for Functional Medicine.) The ACE questionnaire assesses exposure to events like emotional, physical, and sexual abuse, a mother treated violently, parental separation or divorce, drug use, and emotional and physical neglect. The more adverse childhood experiences you've experienced, the higher your score.

When I share this questionnaire with you in a later chapter, you'll have a chance to discover your own score, and you'll learn that six is a high score. With higher ACE scores, both the psyche and the body become dysregulated, and the risk increases for midlife chronic disease, mental illness, violence, and being a victim of violence. People with an ACE score of six or higher are at risk of their life span being curtailed by twenty years. We have increased risk for at least twenty-one autoimmune diseases including celiac, rheumatoid arthritis, diabetes, and irritable bowel disease.[4] Higher ACE scores create physiological strain, heart disease, high blood sugar, cancer, and strokes.

In women in particular, a high ACE score predicts autoimmune disease, which we suspect is due to toxic stress on the person's developing brain in childhood that shows up later in middle age as chronic disease. This same toxic stress switches genes on and off, changing a child's development at the gene level, often putting them into overdrive, hyperarousal, and overfunctioning. For women, every increase in their ACE score is associated with a 20 percent greater likelihood of being hospitalized with an autoimmune disease. Radha and I have a nearly threefold risk of heart disease compared to people with no adverse childhood experiences.[5]

I also didn't think my trauma was affecting me. My trauma was never adequately treated until my fifties. While it's never too late to address trauma, I wasted a lot of time and relationships stuck in trauma mode. I want people to heal much sooner. Once I figured out that I had a significant trauma signature, I looked at the science and was at first discouraged. I wasn't excited about taking antidepressant prescriptions because I knew they were barely effective. Since pills alone don't unwind trauma from the body, I sought to address the root cause, which required looking beyond the usual treatments to somatic-based therapy, Holotropic Breathwork®, and even psychedelic-assisted therapy. I kicked into action and set about clearing trauma from my system with novel approaches, including Hakomi mindfulness-based somatic therapy, an elimination diet, Internal Family Systems therapy, low-dose naltrexone, and quarterly psychedelic medicine. I found these novel treatments so beneficial and healing that I enrolled in three certifications to enable me to offer psychedelic-assisted treatment to my patients and clients. Meanwhile, in my own body, I shifted from a state of pre-autoimmune disease to normal over the past few years, and I will share what worked and what didn't so that you can perform your own self-experiments to find what works best for you too.

Broadening the Definition of Trauma

Because trauma can have such insidious, pervasive, and corrosive effects on the body, mind, and spirit, it's essential that we learn to detect it. That can be easier said than done, both because many of us are culturally

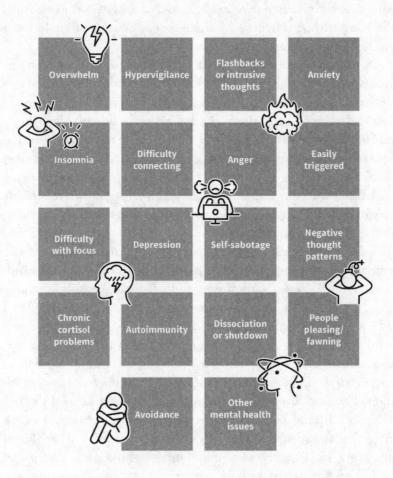

taught to ignore or deny our experiences and because trauma can show up in many ways, some obvious and some not so obvious.

You can think of trauma that persists as an unresolved stress response. I learned a lot about the stress response in my medical training and career. The classic process is that when you're exposed to stress, your body releases adrenaline and cortisol, and then you either take care of business (fight-or-flight, i.e., mobilization toward protection or escape), or you get stuck (freeze, fright, fawn, faint, i.e., incomplete mobilization), meaning you may keep experiencing the original stressor over and over, as if the trauma were still occurring in real time.

Some experts consider stuck, or unresolved, trauma to be a chronic freeze state. Physician and bestselling author Gabor Maté describes trauma as a restriction or constriction in the body and the mental capacity of a person to respond in the present moment from the authentic self.

The stuck path is the topic of this book.

When you get stuck, it can lead to downstream consequences like psychological overwhelm and helplessness, immune problems, neurological difficulties, and hormonal imbalances from the excess adrenaline and cortisol. The immune problems are especially of concern because they may lead to autoimmune conditions, where the body attacks its normal tissues.

I did not learn enough about trauma and unresolved stress responses in my medical training, nor in my twenty-five years of practicing medicine. Yet, as I embarked on my own healing journey and started to ask my patients routinely about trauma, I was surprised to discover how many people were on that stuck path.

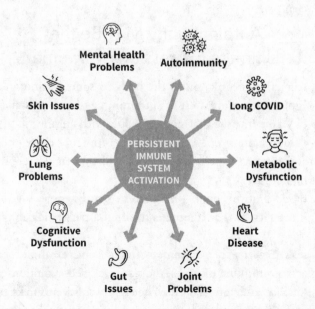

I too was stuck. It's taken me a few decades to realize that the reason I have struggled so much with toxic stress and cortisol is because I was addicted to my body's own stress hormones, trapped in a self-perpetuating loop, in near-constant flight mode, sometimes freeze or fawn, almost never fight. I developed addictive patterns with behaviors that release dopamine, like overworking and overfunctioning in relationships. I craved high-pressure situations and felt bored if there wasn't a lot of tension at the workplace or home. I had a chronic pattern of high conflict in my relationships. I had trouble relaxing and sitting still—I was always on the go. I constantly overscheduled myself. All this, combined with porous boundaries, led to near perpetual cycles of saying yes, then feeling depleted. Until, that is, I started to see the cycle, get help, and change it.

It was only in the last few years that I realized this was no way to live. It's not normal to thrive or succeed in chaos, to stay so busy most of the time, to have trust issues, to feel guilty about resting, or to be so self-reliant that I don't ask for help even when I am completely beyond my capacity. It's exhausting and accelerates aging. It robs you not just of healthspan but also joyspan. But to change what was a subconscious, autonomic process, I had to see and then consciously address it. I had to stop the flight. And that required naming it: trauma.

Autoimmunity May Be the Ultimate Expression of Trauma

Trauma triggers dysregulation in the body in some but not all people. The dysregulation can manifest as autoimmune disease in some but not all people. While it's true that not all people with autoimmunity have a history of trauma, most do. Autoimmunity is the root cause of one hundred chronic illnesses experienced by men and women alike, and women suffer at higher rates.

The big idea of this book—the pattern that I kept seeing in my patients and myself—is that trauma is so often a trigger for autoimmune disease.

Andrea's experience is common and a good example of trauma and classic autoimmune disease. Andrea developed symptoms of autoimmune disease after pregnancy. When she was seven weeks pregnant at age thirty-three, her late husband developed severe headaches. The

shocking diagnosis was a brain tumor, leading to multiple cranioto-
mies, radiation, chemotherapy, and valiant efforts to save his life. Andrea's pregnancy was sidelined by the hardship, medical trauma, and
unending toxic stress. Would her husband survive long enough to meet
their baby? Andrea was in a high gear of overfunctioning that took years
to turn down. It's difficult for her to pinpoint when her autoimmune
symptoms began—was it the unexplained weight loss in pregnancy that
still resulted in birthing a healthy eight-and-a-half-pound baby? Fitting
into her skinny jeans at two weeks postpartum? The hardship wreaked
havoc on her postpartum body, and she experienced a thickening—a
sensation of full-body swelling—that she now thinks of as an inflammatory film. She felt like an alien in her own skin. She had puffiness
under her eyes that no amount of cucumber compresses could remedy,
a sign of wayward inflammation. Eventually, she was diagnosed with
Hashimoto's thyroiditis, the most prevalent autoimmune disease of the
thyroid—and rates of Hashimoto's been increasing for the last few decades.[6] Hashimoto's is eight to ten times more common in women than
men, although men are also affected, and the increased demands of pregnancy contribute to the initial experience of autoimmune thyroid disease
in many women.[7] For Andrea, we can measure her autoimmune activity
by checking the blood level of thyroid peroxidase antibodies (described
further in chapter 7), a type of antibody that targets her normal thyroid
tissue, to assess her self-attack.

When we look at cases of autoimmune disease with root cause
analysis, we consistently find a perfect storm of three factors: genetic
susceptibility, increased intestinal permeability (a condition in which a
person's gut allows more water and nutrients through the cells, i.e., they
leak), and a trigger. Andrea exemplified all three. The trigger can be and
often is trauma. For trauma to trigger, it does not have to be cataclysmic
"big *T*" trauma; it can be just as easily subtle, quiet, minor, or insidious
"little *t*" trauma.

Once I connected trauma and autoimmune disease in my own healing journey, and began to see staggering results with my patients, I knew
I needed to share my work with readers everywhere who are frustrated
and suffering. *The Autoimmune Cure* shares the eating, sleeping, therapy, supplement, and alternative (think MDMA or low-dose naltrexone,
maybe even orgasmic meditation) protocol for people who want to reset
their immune systems and heal autoimmune disorders that come about

"BIG *T*" VERSUS "LITTLE *T*" TRAUMA

"Big *T*" trauma refers to a sudden cataclysmic event that nearly all people consider to be serious, such as a car crash, war, rape, or sudden loss of a loved one, like my friend who just lost her mother to a heart attack and didn't have a chance to say goodbye. "Little *t*" trauma refers to the distressing events that still affect us personally but vary in scope from one person to another, such as a significant breakup, emotional misattunement, or loss of a pet.

We all have varying capacities to manage both "big *T*" and "little *t*" trauma, so it's important to focus on how an individual is impacted by the event rather than the event itself. Both types of trauma can lead to post-traumatic stress disorder, described more fully in chapter 1.

from a variety of triggers, with a focus on this trauma. If you have autoimmune disease, this book is for you, even if you don't feel you've experienced significant trauma. If you have a mysterious illness that has yet to be diagnosed but involves some of the common autoimmune symptoms, like joint aches and fatigue, this book is for you. If someone you love is suffering with autoimmune disease or a mysterious illness, this book is for you, as it will help you think more broadly and support your loved one in their quest for health and healing.

I weave information about my own health and practices into my books and conversations because my life is an n-of-1 experiment, and your life is too, whether you realize it or not, whether you direct your experiments or not. N-of-1 experiments are on the increase because they are easy to perform and give you information that is unique to you since you serve as your own "control" (i.e., reference point).[8] In this book, I will take you by the hand and show you what has been most effective for me, connecting the dots between my psychology and my physiology, including through mind-body therapy like Hakomi; trauma-informed care; practices such as Holotropic Breathwork® that help you enter a healing state of consciousness; emerging technologies to track my physiology, like microbiome testing, continuous glucose monitoring, use of a ring wearable, and tracking heart rate variability; new applications of old medications that can act as immunomodulators, such as low-dose naltrexone; and therapeutic use of psychedelic medicine.

While I've figured out a lot that is right for my health and for the health of others over my career, I'm an eternal student with plenty to learn in terms of being more present and creating healing and wholeness. This journey, described in and motivated by this book, has intertwined learning and healing. As each aspect of my self and my trauma came into the light, I would learn how to release my imperfections, which in turn would teach me to become more present in my wholeness. The act of writing this book is a part of this learning-healing cycle, and I offer it as an invitation to learn together so that we can heal together.

In my books, I write about my practices and experiences not only to share these n-of-1 experiments that might help others and myself but also to connect with others who suffer similarly and need help. Health information is private, and most doctors are indoctrinated during medical training to avoid disclosing anything personal. However, when we bring our secrets and most private information, including trauma, into the light of day, we create space for other people to feel more accepted for what they are working with in life, particularly trauma, and notably the trauma of oppression.

In this book, you'll hear about people who struggle with trauma and how many of them have found their trauma to be a trigger for autoimmune disease or pre-autoimmune disease. This book is intended to be for everyone, regardless of sex, gender, and race. Even so, it's not generic; each person's unique identity comes with an individual physiology that requires personalized understanding, which is made available through study, insight, and vulnerability. This book may help you access your vulnerability, because vulnerability can be a source of protection for us and others. Brené Brown adds: "Vulnerability is the only bridge we have to build connections with others."[9]

I'm introducing this information in this way, through the stories of myself and others, because we need greater communication, explicitness, and consent with the issue of trauma and how it impacts health. For example, if I had known that antidepressants are barely more effective than placebo for trauma, I never would have consented. That's the level of consent that we need to bring to all of medicine, whether that is trauma-informed care or prescriptions for autoimmune disease and immunosuppression. If you've experienced difficult and emotionally painful moments in life and gone to a therapist to talk about it, were you informed that only about one in three people benefit from therapy? Probably not. That's where precision medicine and n-of-1 experiments can be so helpful, because what's true for a large population is only a guide; it's not necessarily true for the individual,[10] and what's true for the individual is not necessarily true for the population.[11]

This book is about how to measure your own level of trauma, assess whether it is causing dysregulation in your body, reprogram, and then reintegrate as a better whole. Resolving my own trauma has helped me land in the present moment with awareness, to be both accepting of and astonished by what is. Now my hope is to share the gift of trauma resolution with you and others. It evokes what my friend Heather shared with me recently, a teaching she paraphrased from psychologist and medical anthropologist Alberto Villoldo: *When we understand we are on a mythic journey, everything changes; we see that everything in our lives is to teach us and heal us for our higher purpose.* I have come to understand my trauma as pointing me toward a mythic journey, and this book is about that process for all of us.

PART 1

··

DECONSTRUCTING
THE PATTERN
Autoimmunity, Trauma, and Hormones

CHAPTER 1

The Autoimmunity Epidemic

You were a disease without name, I was a body gone flame.

—MEGHAN O'ROURKE, "IDIOPATHIC ILLNESS," *SUN IN DAYS*

utoimmune disease affects about one in ten of the world population, and prevalence rates are markedly increasing around the globe. In the United States, twenty-four million people are diagnosed with autoimmune illness. However, these numbers are conservative and represent only the people who *already know* they have autoimmune disease, a complex condition in which the body's immune system mistakes its own healthy tissue as foreign and attacks it. There are people who have a pre-disease state of autoimmune disease that doesn't quite meet diagnostic criteria. There are also people who suffer with symptoms of autoimmune disease and just muscle through it without seeking a diagnosis, chalking it up to aging or hormones or perhaps assume the symptoms are psychosomatic.

This is where conventional medicine can fail the individual, such that the average person with autoimmune disease sees four doctors over three years before they even receive a diagnosis. One woman I care for has spent more than $200,000 in extensive laboratory tests over the past year and still hasn't received a diagnosis yet is being treated with a toxic medication called colchicine, used for autoimmune disease! The problem is that conventional medicine treats symptoms, whereas the type of medicine that I practice addresses and aims to resolve root causes.

I met Kristina at a yoga studio in Northern California. Her regular yoga and meditation practice kept her body, mind, and spirit supple, but in her forties she started to develop profound knee pain and a feeling of crackling, like gravel, in her elbows. Her primary care doctor ran a few tests, told her it looked like rheumatoid arthritis, and referred her to see a rheumatologist. While waiting eight months for an appointment with the specialist, she reached out to me for a consultation.

Rheumatoid arthritis is an autoimmune, chronic inflammatory disorder that affects several joints. The body's immune system attacks the joints and sometimes internal organs. As a result of autoimmune attack by the dysregulated immune system, people with rheumatoid arthritis suffer with painful swelling of the joints, erosion of the bone, and changes in the shape (sometimes deformity) of the joint.

As I took her history, I learned that Kristina had suffered a toxic betrayal in the two years prior to her symptoms. Her husband had an affair with her best friend, which Kristina discovered and then confronted them. Her symptoms began silently, or so she thought.

Kristina's autoimmune attack of her healthy joints increased steadily until her symptoms could no longer be ignored. After her rheumatologist diagnosed her with rheumatoid arthritis, he told her that there's no cure but that medication can slow the progression. As Kristina reflected on the immune effects of the situation, she recalled the sense of shame that she experienced internally. She explained to me, "Not only was life painful (heartbreak), but I was experiencing shame (within the spiritual community)." She was able to heal by letting go of the toxic relationships and dynamics driving her shame and by practicing several of the methods in this book. With time and work, her inflammation resolved, and her symptoms mostly disappeared.

Beyond the one in ten people like Kristina who are diagnosed with autoimmune disease, more people are undiagnosed, misdiagnosed, or not yet diagnosed. They suffer from mysterious symptoms like severe fatigue, brain fog, aches and pains, tingling and numbness, stubborn weight gain and fluid retention (or weight loss like Kristina did), abdominal pain and digestive problems, swollen glands, anxiety and depression, hair loss and insomnia—and don't know that their imbalanced immune system is at the root of their symptoms. When the body's immune system attacks healthy tissues, the most common result is chronic inflammation in different parts of the body, like in your thyroid, hands, or abdomen; the body part depends on the type of autoimmune disease affecting the person. Blood tests that look for autoantibodies, which your immune system may make against your normal tissue, can help diagnose these conditions.

We Don't Track Autoimmune Disease Correctly

The problem of the exponentially rising rate of autoimmune disease further compounds when you consider that we do not track the rate of autoimmune disease systematically here in the United States. There is no official governmental bean counter in charge of autoimmune numbers and no mechanism to collect data about prevalence and incidence of autoimmune disease.

The National Institutes of Health hasn't updated their figures from 2005 when they stated that twenty-four million Americans are affected,[1] though others peg the prevalence higher at fifty million, and sometimes include people with autoantibodies who don't yet have a diagnosis—people like me with positive antibodies against the nucleus of cells, called antinuclear antibodies (ANA) but no clear diagnosis. That's considered pre-autoimmune or latent disease, and the blood test can be positive for seven to fourteen years prior to diagnosis. That's an important opportunity to address the root causes and prevent or reverse the condition, which is what I do as a physician, as do many clinicians like me. We use leading indicators to care for our patients, and they may foretell future disease years before symptoms or a diagnosis.

We are great at tracking infection and cancer, but not whether you have a blood test showing that you have antibodies against your normal tissue and are in the process of destroying that tissue. When we have a match between the antibody and the tissue being attacked, that represents strong evidence that the disease is autoimmune—for example, self-produced antibodies against the thyroid in Hashimoto's thyroiditis or against an enzyme called glutamic acid decarboxylase (GAD) in type 1 diabetes. (You'll read examples of cases of both of these types of autoimmune disease later in the book.) There are so many different autoimmune conditions that academic physicians and policymakers have not yet reached a consensus about the full list of what they are, and some conditions have stronger evidence of autoimmunity than others.

How do we collect accurate data about problems that are not clearly defined? Sadly, that's the current state of affairs with autoimmune disease. Some researchers have noted that autoimmune disease is rising, particularly in places where children are exposed to fewer germs, such as in industrialized countries like the United States and United Kingdom. (Known as the hygiene hypothesis, the idea is that improved sanitation over the past century or so has limited children's exposure to germs and infections—exposures that help a healthy immune system to develop.) Normally, or so the hypothesis goes, immune coaching with germs helps the body learn how to tell the difference between harmful and harmless substances that may trigger autoimmune and allergic diseases, including asthma. Less exposure to germs means less coaching of the immune system and, voilà, more autoimmunity and allergies.

Or you might wonder if the rising rates of autoimmune disease is due to increased diagnosis and reporting. We don't know, but we do know that certain autoantibodies, made by a type of immune cell, are increasing in the US population. The National Institute of Environmental Health Sciences in Durham, North Carolina, analyzed blood from fourteen thousand people over the past twenty-five years for antinuclear antibodies, which are antibodies that your body makes against the normal nucleus of your cells. The earliest samples showed that 11 percent of people were positive for antinuclear antibodies, and the most recent samples showed that 16 percent were positive. The greatest increases occurred in men, non-Hispanic whites, and adolescents—the prevalence tripled in teenagers from 1988 to 2012. This is alarming, and something must be done to address the tsunami of autoimmune attack that is coming our way. Do you know if you have antinuclear antibodies? I didn't in 2012, but I do now, as I'll explain later.

Physicians are less helpful than you might expect when it comes to early intervention or treatment, as conventional clinicians are sometimes only vaguely aware of what is happening in a patient's body in the years prior to a diagnosis. Conventional medicine regularly fails to heal individuals whose symptoms and lab tests don't point to an obvious diagnosis or a clear treatment path. There is another way: a solution based on addressing the root causes of autoimmune disease, one by one. If you're one of the twenty-four million Americans struggling with autoimmune disease, I invite you to roll up your sleeves with me so that we can address the foundation of your disease. If you're one of the hundreds of millions of people facing strange symptoms and chronic inflammation, and you're not sure what's causing it all, this book is for you too. I've helped hundreds of people improve or heal autoimmune symptoms, and I know you can find relief with this program too.

What Is Autoimmune Disease?

The function of the immune system is to protect your body from foreign invasion, such as by viruses or bacteria. The primary strategy that your immune system uses is to produce antibodies, which are like guards that protect you from an invader. For people with a healthy and balanced immune system, these antibodies correctly identify foreign invaders, like a cold virus brought home by your preschooler or a splinter in your finger, and as a rule, they do not attack the cells of your own body.

Autoimmune disease is a complex disorder in which multiple genetic and environmental factors collide. Many issues are intertwined, but the key triad that leads to autoimmunity are heredity, increased intestinal permeability (so-called leaky gut), and then a trigger. These three factors interact with the immune system positively or negatively, and ultimately initiate the cascade of events leading to autoimmune disease. Triggers can vary but range from trauma and toxic stress to infection, from poor dietary choices to big hormonal shifts like pregnancy or perimenopause.

My approach, which you will learn in this book, is a personalized one that leans heavily on lifestyle medicine for the larger and more comprehensive solution. If lifestyle problems got you into trouble with autoimmunity, I imagine that lifestyle medicine can help you get out of it. As our deeper understanding of the interaction factors improves, we are able to formulate more customized treatments to address the root cause of an individual's autoimmunity.

What autoimmune diseases all have in common is that the immune system loses its ability to correctly separate foreign ("non self") from self.

When immune cells make this mistake and attack cells they are supposed to protect, you may develop autoimmune disease. Think of it as the following: the immune system develops a case of mistaken identity.

As a clinician, I can measure the level of self-attack in the blood by tracking *autoantibodies*. As mentioned, these are antibodies against your own healthy tissues, like an enzyme in the thyroid known as thyroid peroxidase or, as we found in Kristina, rheumatoid factor, proteins made by the immune system that can attack your joints in rheumatoid arthritis or Sjögren's syndrome and can be used to pinpoint the diagnosis.

Put into medical language, autoimmune disease is a broad category of related disorders in which the immune system attacks self tissues.[2] When the immune system attacks its own body's cells, the consequence is a form of civil war, and symptoms can range from nuisance to profoundly disabling.

If you have an autoimmune diagnosis, you know that the list of potential problems is long and continues to grow past one hundred potential diagnoses: Hashimoto's thyroiditis, multiple sclerosis, type 1 diabetes, lupus, psoriasis, Crohn's disease, ulcerative colitis, etc.

The Growing Autoimmune List

When I was in medical school, the list of autoimmune diseases was short: lupus, inflammatory bowel disease like Crohn's disease or ulcerative colitis, Sjögren's, type 1 diabetes, multiple sclerosis, and Hashimoto's.

Now the autoimmune list has grown exponentially, along with the number of people affected by it. There are more than one hundred known autoimmune conditions. Why is the prevalence of immune disorganization and dysregulation increasing? Most scientists believe that rates have accelerated because the underlying triggers have accelerated, including stress, poor or inflammatory diet, lack of exercise, insufficient sleep, environmental toxins, and trauma. Skeptics may think this is a marketing ploy to sell supplements, but science disagrees.

Up to fifty million Americans have a disease characterized by immune dysregulation. Symptoms can be mysterious, ranging from joint pain and skin problems to swollen glands and gut issues. Many people have latent or pre-disease that can be present for seven to fourteen years prior to diagnosis, and before anyone, including you, knows what's actually going on.

In my opinion, as we define "autoimmune disease" as "when the immune system gets confused and attacks normal tissue," we might potentially expand the definition to include other conditions: certain forms of heart disease, migraines, irritable bowel disease, chronic Lyme disease, migraines, breast implant illness, and endometriosis are now considered autoimmune. We will explore these conditions in the book as well.

Post-COVID syndrome is now considered an autoimmune disease, or to be an infectious trigger of a future autoimmune disease. In some people, the disease involves a severe inflammatory response in the lungs, the liver, the kidneys, and even the brain. This was initially thought to be due to damage from the virus, but the pattern does not seem to be like other similar viral infections, so investigators have proposed that COVID may be an autoimmune reaction in vulnerable individuals.[3] However, we may not have the full picture for some time since COVID is still so new and we are still clarifying the connection between COVID and autoimmunity.

Root Causes of Autoimmune Disease

As autoimmune disease has skyrocketed in prevalence,[4] our understanding of the root causes continues to expand but is not yet definitive. We know the key factors that interact to cause autoimmune disease, including genetics, environmental exposures, aging, hormones, psychology, gut, and immune function.[5] When you look at the concordance of autoimmune disease in twins, the rates are 12 to 67 percent, meaning there's quite a bit of variation with high heritability for some conditions (type 1 diabetes) and less for others (rheumatoid arthritis or scleroderma).[6] Big hormonal shifts like puberty, pregnancy, perimenopause, and male hypogonadism (low testosterone) can be associated with a greater risk of autoimmune disease.[7]

Most of us clinicians who practice medicine don't think of autoimmune disease as a collection of one hundred–plus diverse and unrelated conditions, but instead think of it as primarily a single problem with many variations depending on how your genes interact with the envi-

THE MOST COMMON AUTOIMMUNE DISEASES

According to the Autoimmune Registry, the most common autoimmune diseases are the following.[8]

- Rheumatoid arthritis—a chronic inflammatory condition in which the immune system attacks the joints, particularly of the hands and feet.
- Hashimoto's thyroiditis—a condition in which the immune system attacks the thyroid gland in the neck.
- Celiac disease—an immune reaction to eating gluten, a protein in wheat, barley, and rye. It leads to inflammation and damage of the small intestine and may prevent absorption of nutrients.
- Graves' disease—an immune system disorder of the thyroid that leads to overproduction of thyroid hormones.
- Diabetes mellitus, type 1—a chronic condition in which the immune system attacks the pancreas gland, so that the cells can no longer produce enough insulin.
- Vitiligo—a condition that leads to loss of skin color in patches on any part of the body.
- Rheumatic fever—a disease that results from insufficiently treated strep throat or scarlet fever, causing inflammation of the heart, blood vessels, and joints.
- Pernicious anemia/atrophic gastritis—an autoimmune disease that prevents your body from absorbing vitamin B12. Symptoms include weakness and fatigue and, if untreated, may cause heart and nerve damage.
- Alopecia areata—a condition in which the immune system attacks hair follicles, leading to one or more circular bald patches.
- Immune thrombocytopenic purpura—a condition that occurs when the immune system attacks platelets by mistake, and the resulting low levels of platelets lead to increased bleeding. Symptoms include easy bruising, bleeding, and pinpoint-sized red/purple spots on the lower legs.
- Post-COVID syndrome (or "long COVID")—a condition that occurs in up to half of cases of COVID-19 infection and can affect a person for months to years. Data is primarily anecdotal and requires more rigorous scientific inquiry. Symptoms include fatigue, an unpredictable flare-and-remission pattern of recurrence, and brain fog.

ronment and cause an imbalanced immune system and inflammation. That's what the science suggests.

What is triggering the increase in autoimmunity? Triggers are less clear, but usually something sets off the gene/environment problem, like trauma. "Trauma" is derived from Greek and, as we will explore in the next few chapters, refers to a wound that may hurt you not just psychologically but also physically. It is a form of toxic stress that may halt the healthy development of your emotional, immune, neurological, and hormonal systems. As Gabor Maté, MD, describes, "Trauma is not what happens to you, it's what happens inside you as a result of what happened to you. Trauma is that scarring that makes you less flexible, more rigid, less feeling and more defended."

Did Kristina's trauma kick off the self-attack of her knee and elbows? We don't know for sure, but I believe it did, that her wounding left specific tissues less resilient and more vulnerable to self-attack of autoimmunity.

Increasingly, we understand that trauma plays a greater role than previously understood in your physical health. Studies show that up to 80 percent of patients with autoimmune disease experience significant emotional stress before disease onset.[9] What gives? Unhealthy levels of stress may impair the immune system and increase your future risk of autoimmune disease. I see this routinely in my medical practice.

Take the 9/11 terrorist bombings as an example. There are 41,656 people enrolled in the World Trade Center Health Registry, including first responders and community members. In the years following the 9/11 exposure, first responders with dust cloud exposure had an 85 percent higher risk of systemic autoimmune disease. People with PTSD had a 250 percent greater risk of systemic autoimmune disease. Which diseases? The most common are rheumatoid arthritis ($n = 75$), Sjögren's syndrome ($n = 23$), systemic lupus erythematosus ($n = 20$), myositis ($n = 9$), mixed connective tissue disease ($n = 7$), and scleroderma ($n = 4$).[10] While this is not definitive evidence that trauma causes autoimmune disease, it is strong evidence in favor of the theory.

What about military personnel? We now know from the Millennium Cohort, a large study of 120,572 active-duty service members in the United States followed for at least five years, that PTSD raises the risk of autoimmune disease by 58 percent compared to no history of

PTSD.[11] The conditions studied included rheumatoid arthritis, systemic lupus erythematosus, inflammatory bowel diseases, and multiple sclerosis. The Millenium Cohort study confirmed a prior study of 666,289 Iraq and Afghanistan veterans showing that PTSD, diagnosed in 31 percent, is associated with a twofold greater risk of autoimmune disease. While women suffer more with autoimmune disease than men, the magnitude of PTSD-associated risk of autoimmune disease was similar in men and women.

The takeaway is that while we focus on the *psychiatric* risk of toxic stress, particularly in veterans and other people who experience trauma, we need to be thinking more about the *physical* risk they face related to stress disorders, including autoimmune disease. We separate mental from physical health, when in fact they are two sides of the same coin. How then is trauma exposure connected to other triggers in one's lifestyle, like food and air quality, changes in hormones and the nervous system, altered immune function and autoimmunity, and even the way genes talk to the body? The more we understand, the more we can provide informative, mitigative, and transformative strategies to heal.

View from My Medical Office

What I'm seeing in my medical office at Thomas Jefferson University—where I work as a physician offering a whole health approach as the director of precision medicine—is that my schedule is filled with people who suffer with autoimmune disease. The most common condition that I see is autoimmune thyroid disease. Others have type 1 diabetes diagnosed right at menopause. Quite a few have psoriasis or celiac or ulcerative colitis or Crohn's disease or rheumatoid arthritis. Some have conditions that only some doctors, like myself, consider to be autoimmune, such as coronary heart disease in their forties, endometriosis, migraines, fibromyalgia, or irritable bowel syndrome.

What surprises me is that when I ask about trauma, many of my autoimmune patients tell me about significant exposures. While I certainly have my share of patients with post-traumatic stress disorder (PTSD) after combat in the military, most of them have a more common and insidious experience of toxic stress, such as adverse childhood experiences like physical or sexual abuse, a parent who drank too much and was

DEPRESSION: IMMUNE ATTACK?

Depression comes in many forms. What if depression is actually an inflammation disorder in the body that begins in the gut and then seeps into the brain? What if trauma has a similar effect? Medical doctors and scientists previously believed that depression, or major depressive disorder in medical language, was simply an imbalance of brain chemicals like serotonin, norepinephrine, and dopamine—and that these neurotransmitters needed adjustment individually, sometimes in isolation with a drug that affects serotonin (a selective serotonin reuptake inhibitor, like fluoxetine or sertraline), or a combination (a selective serotonin norepinephrine reuptake inhibitor, like duloxetine or escitalopram). But these medications don't work that well. For duloxetine (trade name Cymbalta), one has to treat six to nine people in order for one person to benefit.[12] That means upward of millions of people globally are taking antidepressants with little to no benefit. Humanity needs a better way.

Physicians and scientists increasingly believe that depression, along with other psychiatric illnesses, may be a result of immune dysregulation involving the central nervous system.[13] Some experts even suggest that depression is a form of allergy where the immune system attacks healthy tissue.[14] People with depression, like Justin, whom you'll meet in chapter 12, experience a greater risk of autoimmune disease compared to people without a history of depression. The higher risk of autoimmune disease occurs in the first year after the onset of depression. The effect is once again bidirectional: up to half of people with autoimmune disease show impaired quality of life and depressive symptoms.

Our advances in neuroscience are astonishing, yet they fall short in benefiting people who suffer with trauma and dysregulation. When you consider the state of mental health in our country and globally, psychiatry is the only specialty in which the prevalence of illness is increasing over time, unlike other fields, like cardiology or urology.[15] We need better tools to navigate mental health in collaboration with patients, as well as the broader context in which mental health occurs, including the role of diet, trauma, exercise, gut function, toxic exposure, autoimmunity, spiritual difficulties, and prolonged grief.

mean, or neglect. Or a loved one who died during the pandemic. Or ancestral trauma related to parents who survived something horrible, like the Holocaust or a Japanese internment camp or racism. One woman in her forties with psoriasis had birth trauma, which significantly worsened her symptoms of itchy rash, scaly patches, and thickened plaques on her hands and elbows. You'll get to know several of these patients throughout this book.

As I started to link autoimmunity and trauma, I realized there's an important opportunity for us to broaden the definition of trauma and the stress response it creates in the body. More importantly, I discovered that my twenty-five years of practicing medicine was insufficient at addressing trauma. As I wrote this book, I was surprised to find that a fight with my family could raise my resting heart rate from sixty to ninety beats per minute, and raise my fasting blood sugar to a similar extent. There were neurobiological effects from my psychosocial environment, and I hadn't realized how much psychosocial events were causing problems with my physiology, particularly my immune, neurological, and hormone systems. As part of the preparation for this book, I've taken a deep dive into what it feels like *in my body* to be regulated versus dysregulated, and I've learned how to regulate myself with breathwork and other means. I've experimented with microbiome modulation and psychedelic-assisted therapy, and completed comprehensive training in mindfulness-based somatic therapy. The net result is that I'm regulated more of the time, and I'm less tolerant of the people and experiences that cause dysregulation for me. Why does this matter? We assume that an elevated resting heart rate or blood pressure or blood sugar is a bad thing to be fixed—maybe with a prescription medication—but what if we open the aperture and recognize that many of these indicators could be telling us a more important story about persistent trauma that keeps getting reactivated, or even new trauma exposures that we don't yet think of as trauma?

If you are someone who suffers from autoimmune disease, or are heading in that direction, or know someone with autoimmune disease, I want you to understand the connection between autoimmunity and trauma so that you can start to unlock the trauma response that may be driving some or maybe even most of your autoimmune symptoms. You don't have to be a veteran with flashbacks to benefit from what I'm providing in this book. At this point in our polarized and divided world, most of us have experienced trauma in some way, shape, or form, and the question is whether it might still be embedded in your system, driving nagging and sometimes disabling symptoms that prevent you from the fullest expression of your life.

A Vicious Cycle of Autoimmune Disease

Toxic stress can trigger disease, but a diagnosis of autoimmune disease often creates another layer of stress in patients, causing a vicious cycle. Bathed in the stress-related hormones like adrenaline and cortisol that alter or amplify immune system weapons like cytokines (small proteins secreted by cells in the immune system that can cause inflammation), you may be putting yourself at unnecessary risk of worsening immune regulation and autoimmune disease.

It is possible to break the vicious cycle. I taught myself and my patients how to do it, after decades of struggling with the default factory setting of high stress levels. Sometimes a reality check such as a grim diagnosis finally gets you to change.

The first step is to understand the pattern that leads to autoimmune disease in a way that weaves together what we know and don't know, including the role of trauma, and that is what we will cover in Part 1 of this book. You'll learn about the immune system and how it gets out of balance from certain stressors (e.g., how your childhood neglect or divorce or birthing experience got under your skin and set up dysregulation in your present life).

The second step is to heal, to reintegrate your parts into a state of wholeness, to build resilience, and that is what we will cover in Part 2 of this book. Briefly, this process involves new transformative principles often missing in conventional medicine, like safety, interaction, tracking, regulating, resourcing, and collaboration. In the top-down, authoritative practice of medicine, the body is a problem to be fixed by the expert, the doctor. It's a cookie-cutter approach that works in an emergency, but not for chronic disease. I learned how to do it, but found it missed the mark. Now I reject the approach when caring for people with chronic disease. Of course, it can be helpful when you're overwhelmed by a diagnosis of cancer or a broken bone, but for chronic illness such as autoimmune disease, it is not sufficiently collaborative and considering of your unique needs.

One of my patients with autoimmune disease, a man in his mid-twenties with Hashimoto's, came to me on Synthroid, which was prescribed by his previous physician with minimal conversation about the risks, benefits, and alternatives. As we got to know each other, I learned that he was experiencing cold hands and it was affecting his work in fitness. He had a history of exposure to radiation from childhood, which may have been a potential trigger for his Hashimoto's thyroiditis. He also had childhood trauma and an adverse childhood experience score of four. Together we decided to focus on rebuilding his gut health and to add a small dose of T3 to his Synthroid. We worked on tension patterns in his trapezius, shoulders, and the nerve bundle from his chest to his arms to identify areas that needed nourishment. We changed the pillows for sleep. His symptoms are 90 percent better, not because of top-down directives but from our ongoing conversation and experiments about how we can support his optimal health and resilience.

My greatest hope is that you will use this book to trust your experience, to change without an agenda or force, and to feel fully empowered to transform as you are ready. In Part 2, you will reconnect to your self-knowledge, inherent wisdom of the body, and activate self-healing. This is assisted self-study, to remember how to feel the flow of your true internal experience.

What to Do When You're Diagnosed with (or Suspect You Have) an Autoimmune Disease

Those with autoimmune disease are encouraged to calm down, take it easy, and consider a range of pharmaceuticals that mimic stress hormones—steroids, immunosuppressive drugs, even pills for anxiety, depression, sleep, and pain. We are told there is nothing we can do about the course of autoimmunity, but I disagree. Conventional medicine groups symptoms together in a way that allows the application of a pharmaceutical to slow down the inevitable decline in health resulting from autoimmune disease, but this process disregards root cause in favor of symptom management, and potentially disconnects a patient from the empowering role in creating a different reality for themselves.

Most of my patients don't want to take a pill for temporary symptom relief that can cause harm to the body over time. They want a different approach that addresses issues at the root of illness, and that's what I offer you in this book: a lasting solution to autoimmune disease that attends to the root cause of your condition. While autoimmune disease tends to be a chronic condition that you can manage better with the tools in this book, I have seen some cases of patients who have gotten their autoimmune disease in full remission.

Circling Back to Kristina

Were Kristina's symptoms caused by her trauma? We don't know. Certainly, the timing was suggestive. As I'll share with you, her root cause, like in most patients, is likely a perfect storm of genetic vulnerability and environmental triggers (perhaps the severe stress of her marriage ending in infidelity). In later chapters, I'll share the evidence that showed up in her labs: cortisol and estrogen surges, high inflammatory tone, cholesterol problems, heavy metal toxicity. Toxic stress resulting in abnormal cortisol levels has short- and long-term consequences, ranging from gut damage to high blood sugar;[16] autoimmune disease and inflammation;[17] and brain injury, shrinkage, and cognitive impairment[18]—even in healthy women in their forties like Kristina.[19] Her case illustrates why there is such a dramatic increase in autoimmune disease in today's world, related to the rise of a broad array of toxins including diets full of sugar and refined carbohydrates, toxic stress, toxic culture, and other environmental exposures.

Kristina and I worked together to define a personalized blueprint, similar to the one shared in this book, that has led her one year later to be almost entirely free of symptoms and on zero prescription medicine. She worked mindfully with nutrition, lifestyle, and psychedelics to heal her body and spirit. It worked.

No standard autoimmune treatment program acknowledges the link between trauma and autoimmunity. In the rest of Part 1, we will explore the connections between trauma, hormones, and autoimmunity that are so important to understand in order to heal from autoimmunity.

Wrap-Up

I wrote this book about autoimmunity and one of its potential causes, trauma, because causation is commonly overlooked. By reducing or healing toxic lifestyle factors that are scientifically tied to autoimmune attack, you can address the root cause of autoimmune disease and tip the balance back to health. But it goes beyond eating whole foods, drinking filtered water, and prioritizing sleep. We will choose from novel approaches to self-regulation, such as psychedelic breathwork, microbiome restoration, somatic therapy, naltrexone, internal family systems, ketamine-assisted treatment, potentially microdosing "magic mushrooms," and maybe even MDMA-assisted therapy. Of course, the healing modalities that I describe in this book can be beneficial to you, regardless of whether you are currently diagnosed with an autoimmune problem.

When you remove the root cause of imbalances and add in nourishing resources, you can reap what hundreds of my autoimmune patients have gained: resilience, disease remission, and robust health.

CHAPTER 2

Trauma, Hormones, and the Root Cause of Autoimmunity

Trauma produces actual physiological changes, including a recalibration of the brain's alarm system, an increase in stress hormone.

—BESSEL VAN DER KOLK, *THE BODY KEEPS THE SCORE*

Aaron is a thirty-nine-year-old serial entrepreneur who came to me for an executive health consultation at Thomas Jefferson University. His latest obsession was day trading as a way of protecting his growing wealth. Unfortunately for Aaron, it was clear that while the market was down, his symptoms of scalp itch and irritable bowel were going up. One look at the thick, swollen patches on the top of his head, and I could see that he had scalp psoriasis, an autoimmune disease. Even irritable bowel disease, long thought to be a diagnosis of exclusion, is considered autoimmune in some cases, especially the diarrhea type that Aaron experiences.[1]

As physicians, we are trained to use a more traditional approach to solve the problem, offering the latest pharmaceutical products, which only work part of the time because they may not address the root cause. In the type of medicine that I practice, we look at the root causes for autoimmunity. And as I peel back the layers of each patient's story, I often find the lingering biological and emotional effects of trauma, signaling that the root cause may be a prior overwhelming experience. How does this happen? Trauma can combine with genetic vulnerability and other environmental exposures, like unhealthy food and exercise habits, and lead to many chronic conditions, including autoimmune disease. And while a lucky few of us are spared from the type of trauma that can have these effects, we are fortunate to now have access to many solutions that can potentially reverse disease.

In Aaron's case, what was the root cause of his scalp psoriasis and irritable bowel syndrome (IBS) that would sometimes send him racing to the bathroom at inopportune moments? (While this has not yet become standard thinking in conventional medicine, we believe some forms of IBS are autoimmune, as demonstrated first by Mark Pimentel, MD, a gastroenterologist and associate professor of medicine at Cedars-Sinai Medical Center in Los Angeles.) What was setting off Aaron's symptoms? Was he stressed by the volatile economic landscape? Most of us are—in a study of the COVID-19 pandemic, global prevalence of mental health issues is at an all-time high: depression is at 28 percent, anxiety at 27 percent, and psychological distress at 50 percent.[2]

Or was there something from Aaron's past that was connected to his current experience of daily life, an old incident that was stuck in his present suffering? If so, how did an old event get under his skin and trigger his immune system to attack his own cells? Did he need healing from trauma? Was his emotional coping style working for or against him?

When we discussed his history, Aaron didn't mention trauma, which is defined by psychiatrist Bessel van der Kolk, MD, as "not the story of something that happened back then, but the current imprint of that pain, horror, and fear living inside." Instead, Aaron described a relatively normal childhood growing up in Pennsylvania, the third of three children. But as I probed deeper, Aaron started describing traumatic events—as a child, he was physically threatened, he was hit by a parent with a belt, he felt like he had no one to protect him, his parents were separated, his brother was depressed, and his mother was physically hurt by his father more than once.

According to Aaron, these issues were not a big deal. But his body has a different point of view. Trauma was lodged in his body, specifically his psycho-immune-neuro-endocrine, or PINE, system.

The PINE system illustrates the way you respond to your environment. This concept is sometimes described as psychoneuroimmunology, or psycho-neuro-endocrine-immunology. I prefer PINE because it's easier to remember. PINE is a scientific area of study that investigates the bidirectional communication between the mind and its functions, the immune system, the nervous system, the endocrine system, and how they all connect to physical, mental, and spiritual health. You can consider the PINE to be your stress response system. Some of us have a very sensitive PINE system; others, less so.

Think of the PINE system as a tool kit for detecting danger in the external world. Your tool kit draws on the autonomic nervous system, which is the part of the nervous system that controls involuntary activ-

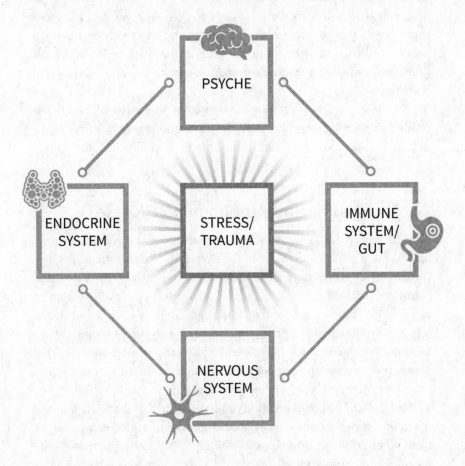

ity, like your heartbeat and breathing. When the system gets harmed by trauma, you may not be able to regulate things like your response to stress, how fast you breathe, and the widening of your blood vessels. As a result, you may fly off the handle under stress, feel anxious or irritable, raise your pulse and blood pressure much higher than is healthy, sleep poorly, and poke holes in the lining of your gut. That can set you up for autoimmune disease to take hold. We believe this cascade of untoward events and effects are at the root of IBS, depression, anxiety, and autoimmune diseases, though the exact mechanisms are still being investigated.[3]

You may not even remember the moment the alarm went off, but your PINE system does. When the stress response system is stuck in the "on" position as a result of overwhelming experiences, your immune, nervous, and endocrine systems are thrown out of whack. In order to heal, you need to revisit the trauma or triggering stress, feel the emotions you began to experience, and fully and truly process them in order to allow your stress response system to move to the "off" position. That's what we mean by completing the trauma and returning to homeostasis.

I'm here to help you. It's my honor, and my life mission. And in the rest of this chapter, we will explore the connections between autoimmunity and trauma, and how we can heal the body and the mind.

Trauma and Autoimmune Disease

Trauma has an academic definition, but then it has a real-life, simplified explanation. It's a moment in time when the PINE system gets dysregulated. It's when your entire body turns on an alarm. When that alarm goes off—in response to the tone of voice of your father before he raged or hit you, or your mother drinking too much alcohol and checking out—your nervous system, your hormones, your immune system, and your psychology kick into overdrive. You record that moment, that alarm, that pattern, so your body can protect you in the future, even in situations where you don't need protection. And the pattern locks.

Your alarm bells can go off because of "little *t*" trauma, such as the death of a pet of a significant relationship, non-life-threatening injuries from a car accident, or emotional abuse. "Little *t*" trauma commonly includes the chronic misattunement that you may experience in your marriage or partnership. Or trauma can be of the "big *T*" variety, which involves sexual violence or life-threatening experience, even if you were not physically harmed. We all have individual capacities to handle toxic stress, known as resilience, so in some ways, the type of trauma matters less than your unique response to it. Research shows definitively that heightened stress can become biologically embedded in the body, which is how we stay stuck in old patterns from moments in childhood and adulthood, both "little *t*" trauma and "big *T*" Trauma.

Once your PINE system is harmed by trauma or Trauma, even smaller daily stressors can affect you more negatively than they would otherwise. This happened to me. In my thirties, I could not understand why life felt so hard. Granted, I had two kids, a busy career, and a mortgage, but I felt too young to feel so stressed most of the time. Looking deeper, I had a cortisol level that was two to three times higher than it should be. My gut was leaky, my hair was falling out, and a blood test showed that I was developing antibodies against my normal tissues, even though I didn't have an official autoimmune diagnosis. After experiencing adversity, I developed a bias toward expecting threats and danger; I lived in a state of fear, because I didn't feel safe and supported. My PINE tool kit was on high alert, searching the environment for signs that I was not safe. These symptoms were the result.

The PINE system was designed to help us respond to the outside world, and we are hardwired by our experiences to greet that world with one of two responses: welcoming or defended. You can think of the "welcoming" response as the default setting. Your interaction with the environment is regulated, and no alarms go off when you meet someone new or encounter a new situation. Your mind, gut, heart, immune, endocrine, and nervous systems tell you that you are safe.

On the other hand, negative experiences as a kid or an adult create the "defended" response. Sigmund Freud, MD, first coined the term "defense mechanisms," which are psychological forms of protection that keep us from dying, usually developed in our family of origin. They don't always make sense, like denial, repression, or projection. They are primitive responses to not feeling safe.

This is how everyday stressors can become toxic and trigger the "defended" response. Just as the environment may not feel safe, leading to heightened defense, your own body may not feel safe, even though it is the place where we are meant to have the most sovereignty. You may become highly sensitive. It's more difficult to trust people and situations. No matter how hard you try, you have trouble relaxing and feeling at ease. By extension, your immune system gets chaotic and becomes overactive, chronically on the alert, and this leads to increased inflammation and sometimes autoimmune disease.

We know and science has shown that stressors experienced as a kid can lead to stress-related illness in middle age. This cause-and-effect relationship makes sense on a biological level.

From a scientific perspective, childhood trauma can substantially affect your health in your thirties and beyond. As an example: when you feel threatened, your adrenaline goes up, then your cortisol. The high cortisol temporarily raises your blood sugar, so you can fight or flee. But if you experienced a lot of stress as a child—such as a parent's messy divorce or abuse—you may feel stressed most of the time even when you're safe, and as a result, your blood sugar may be chronically high.[4] Overall, as we will cover in chapter 3, trauma exposure can lead to a healthy response that includes resolution and return to homeostasis, or balance. However, in vulnerable individuals, trauma exposure may lead to a faulty response that does not resolve and persists as physiological dysregulation. Trauma is a common trigger of the less-than-healthy stress response that leads to future mental, emotional, and physical health problems, including autoimmunity.

At first, Aaron didn't see a relationship between his childhood and his current medical issues, but as I explained the lingering effects of trauma on the body, the pieces started to click into place for him.

Let's take a closer look at the research about how trauma and autoimmunity are intertwined.

Stress System in Overdrive—What Next?

There are four primary ways that you can connect the dots between trauma and autoimmunity: through your psychology, immune system, nervous system, and endocrine (PINE) system. Let's look first at an example involving hormones and the endocrine system, before examining the rest of the PINE system. While the sequence of events is not linear, I find it helpful to think first of them separately, even though these steps overlap and crosstalk.

The Stress Hormones That Don't Resolve

Imagine you get bitten by a dog as a young child and you require stitches to repair the wound. The pain of the experience may be reduced by a caregiver who took care of you, wiped away your tears, and soothed you while the doctor stitched your torn tissues back together.

The high level of stress triggers a cascade of stress hormones in the brain: corticotropin releasing hormone, or CRH, in the hypothalamus, which triggers the release of another hormone known as adrenocorticotropic hormone, ACTH, in the pituitary gland. Then ACTH stimulates the adrenals in the midback to release cortisol.

In this situation, the stress resolves rapidly and completely, and you learn over time to regulate yourself, so the stress hormones don't cause damage. Self-regulation is when you can regulate your PINE system— your psychology, immune system, nerves, and hormones—without intervention from outside, like a parent or therapist. Ideally, your caregiver teaches you how to do it and models the behavior. In this situation, the stress response system remains normal and balanced. Your gut continues to function, your immune system returns to normal, you go back to a healthy hormone level, and your nervous system gets back to baseline.

The single event of a dog bite could be considered a "little *t*" trauma, and the care of a loving adult helps to ameliorate any lasting effects.

Now imagine a worse situation, a deeper Trauma. Consider cumulative trauma. Instead of a onetime dog bite, it's a household member who belittles you or hits you. You feel that pain regularly at home. Add to that financial insecurity or a parent with mental illness or alcohol use disorder, and the problems compound further. The same cascade of CRH, ACTH, and cortisol occurs, but now you've got these stress hormones coursing through your blood more regularly, and the high levels may not completely resolve. The control system for these hormones can become faulty, known as hypothalamic-pituitary-adrenal axis dysregulation.

Your Immune System, Located Mostly in Your Gut, Gets Triggered

When the stress response is stuck in high alert from cumulative trauma, it can shift the problem from your endocrine system to your immune system, located primarily in your gut, underneath the gut lining. When our immune system evolved, most of the threats we faced were germs we ate or drank, so it makes sense that most of the immune battleground is in the gut. Now we face fewer threats—things like parasites, viruses, and bacteria from food and drink. Our greatest threat is external stress and trauma, and our immune system didn't evolve to cope with it. It's how our endocrine system evolved to talk to our gut, and for the chronically stressed, you may view it as a design flaw.

Several problems snowball because of excess exposure to trauma and the ensuing cascade of stress hormones. Trauma disrupts the delicate balance of microbes in your gut so that there are more villains than friends, a problem called dysbiosis. You may lose the microbial diversity that is a hallmark of health.

Over time, the increased stress hormones (mainly CRH) poke holes in your gut,[5] leading to inappropriate stimulation of the immune system and, in some people, conditions such as IBS[6] and perhaps autoimmune disease, but data are somewhat limited.[7] *Nature*, one of our best medical journals, describes how the role of the intestinal permeability can change from arbitrator, like a bouncer outside of a club deciding whom to let in, to provocateur in inflammatory bowel disease.[8] Put another way, you are supposed to have a barrier in the gut that keeps the bad guys (bacteria, viruses, gluten) out, but that barrier can become faulty and let in the bad guys. Too much stress and CRH can poke holes in your tight junctions in the gut, turning the barrier into cheesecloth.

The net result is that your immune system becomes overstimulated by the combination of leaky gut, dysbiosis, and loss of microbial diversity.[9] I'm simplifying a very complex process so that you can understand how to solve it, but in a nutshell, your immune system becomes overwhelmed, sometimes leading to mistakes in separating bad guys from good guys. Your immune system may get *overactivated into autoimmunity*.

Now your hormones and your immune system are out of whack.

Your Nervous System Gets Locked in a Stress Response

While your endocrine and immune systems get pushed past their ability to regulate themselves, the same thing occurs in the nervous system. At its simplest, the nervous system has two components: one that functions under our conscious control (opening the refrigerator), and one that functions without our conscious control (breathing). The latter component, as mentioned earlier, is known as the autonomic nervous system, where emotional material is either dispelled in the sympathetic nervous system or conserved in the parasympathetic nervous system. Ideally, the autonomic nervous system alternates between the sympathetic and parasympathetic branches in a dynamic process that provides support for optimal digestion, immune surveillance, hormone balance, cognition, and sleep.

When the stress response registers in the limbic system and triggers the release of stress hormones, cumulative stressors can cause the sympathetic nervous system to be locked in the "on" position. As a result, many people who experience trauma feel unable to calm down. Trauma disrupts the rhythm and balance between the sympathetic nervous system and parasympathetic nervous system. The parasympathetic nervous system is where regeneration and healing occur, but it can also trigger dissociation and immobilization.

People with embedded trauma are primed to react—becoming hypervigilant, anxious, restless, potentially angry, panicked, or even dissociated. Your body stores the trauma in your brain, stress response, hormonal control system, gut, immune system, and nervous system. All of these parts have peptide receptors that provide access and store memories of emotional information. Trauma is stored as a memory of overwhelming experience in the network.

At this point, your nervous system is in a state of alarm, along with your hormones and immune system. While the trauma may be hidden inside of the body, the wheels are turning toward an untenable situation that can lead to chronic health conditions, as we've discussed. Ultimately, your immune system gets confused and mistakes your own tissue as a foreign invader and goes into attack mode.

Your Psychology Changes

The most common responses psychologically to trauma are known as fight-flight-freeze-fawn, that is, a stress response system in overdrive. When the stress response was first studied almost one hundred years ago, we thought it was simply fight or flight, but now we know that there are other reactions to stress, including the freeze-and-fawn response, which is more common in women and people who are chronically maltreated.

Fight: when you face a perceived threat aggressively
Flight: when you flee from danger
Freeze: when you're unable to move or act against a threat, like a
deer caught in headlights
Fawn: when you behave pleasingly in an effort to avoid conflict

In essence, trauma can cause chronic stress, increased fear, disempowerment, and irritability, often making it difficult to even sleep. Responses can be immediate or delayed, and include a range of symptoms, including nightmares, flashbacks, anxiety, depression, avoidance of emotions or activities associated with the trauma, fatigue, and sleep disruption.

These four stress responses that can link trauma to overactivation of your psycho-immuno-neuro-endocrine system set up susceptible individuals to autoimmune disorders. At some point, you may be able to measure in the blood of an individual who has been through these four steps rising levels of an inappropriate immune response—usually an antibody against normal tissue. This may explain why the escalation of autoimmune disease cannot be explained by genetic factors alone. The role of toxic stress is well demonstrated for some autoimmune diseases more than others, particularly autoimmune type 1 diabetes, multiple sclerosis, and systemic lupus erythematosus.[10] For most autoimmune disease, toxic stress may precede the onset of symptoms like in Kristina's and Aaron's cases, or toxic stress may affect symptoms later on.

Jamming the Thermostat: Trauma and Dysregulation

Trauma may cause your PINE system to become dysregulated—affecting your psychology, mind, gut, heart, hormones, nervous system, and immune system. Dysregulation means your emotional responses are poorly modulated. You respond worse to stress. Dysregulation is common in many of the conditions that I treat as a physician and have experienced myself, like disordered eating and addiction. Some mental health professionals, such as Nicole LePera, PhD, known as the Holistic Psychologist, believe that all mental health disorders may be rooted in dysregulation.

I believe the problem of dysregulation and the wreckage caused by it extend beyond mental health.

Not all childhood trauma causes dysregulation. If you had a loving presence in your life who believed in you and helped you calm down your state of alarm, you're better off—the trauma is less likely to lead to defenses that can color future behavior, relationships, and health.

By contrast, those who were alone with their pain tend to fare the worst. They are bathed not in a nurturing love and understanding, but in a hot stew of stress hormones, like epinephrine, norepinephrine, and cortisol. The body becomes used to those high levels of stress hormones and reestablishes a set point, like a thermostat getting set to a higher heat. Over time, that thermostat can get jammed and not return to the normal temperature. This represents a stress response system that is now stuck and no longer can be adjusted based on the temperature in the room (i.e., the stress that you encounter). Say you get a nasty email or hit a traffic jam, and you overreact. You get hot and stay hot. Normally, anger or frustration should last for ninety seconds, then you cool off, such as in response to a triggering email. If your thermostat doesn't work, it may take you longer to cool down, if you still can.

Many people with trauma develop a dysregulated response to stress, and they see red with even a slight provocation, as if it's a full-tilt alarm. Some view this as high sensitivity. We can measure the dysregulated response psychologically, emotionally, and physically. That's the type of work that I do: I measure the level of dysregulation in my patients

and help create a path to return them to healthy balance. We repair the thermostat. You can measure this dysregulation before or after disease develops, but the sooner you intervene, the easier it is to return to homeostasis, or balance.

How do we measure dysregulation? We can estimate dysregulation of the stress response system by looking at stress hormones. The primary stress hormone is cortisol, made in the adrenal glands of the mid-back. When dysregulation is present, you may have a cortisol level that is too high or low, or even both in the same day. In the gastrointestinal system, we can measure dysregulation as loss of diversity of microbes, imbalances in the types of microbes (known as dysbiosis) and increased intestinal permeability (leaky gut). In the immune system, we can create a white blood cell map or measure levels of chemical messengers like cytokines. In the nervous system, we can look at heart rate variability and vagal tone. You can also assess genetics to see what you might be vulnerable to develop, such as autoimmune diseases and other stress-related conditions. Finally, you can measure how the genes are expressed (show themselves) and how fast you are aging as a result, an area known as epigenetics. Think of your DNA (genetics) as your hardware, and the gene expression (epigenetics) as the software. For example, you may have a brother whose hair went white in his thirties or a grandfather with black hair until his eighties. The expression of genes may explain some of that.

Many people with trauma develop serious health conditions as a result of that jammed thermostat, not realizing the link to trauma. It depends on your genetic vulnerabilities and how they interact with your environment. For Aaron, it's scalp psoriasis and IBS. For others, it might be celiac, autoimmune thyroiditis, or destruction of the pancreas leading to rising blood sugar and diabetes. For a group of ninety-eight mothers pregnant during 9/11 who developed post-traumatic stress disorder (PTSD), it's their level of cortisol, and then the level of cortisol in their babies, according to a research study led by Rachel Yehuda, PhD.[11] For a group of 371 first responders at the World Trade Center, ten genes were downregulated significantly in the people who developed PTSD.[12] For racial minorities, particularly Black people, cumulative trauma can lead to intergenerational depression that is often more severe, longer in duration, and more likely to be disabling.[13]

Gradient from Health to Disease: Can We Recognize Altered Pathways Earlier?

Functional medicine clinicians are detectives who tend to look more deeply at autoimmune conditions from a systems biology perspective and therefore may order more tests than in mainstream medicine. Some of my colleagues believe that this way of practicing is simply overutilization of testing, but if you have an autoimmune disease, you may disagree. Even our conventional, peer-reviewed journals like the *Journal of the American Medical Association* (*JAMA*) are publishing articles that document "pre-disease" (i.e., pre-autoimmune disease) and how it can be measured in the blood potentially years before a diagnosis of autoimmune disease.

In one study from Sweden, a group of 106,464 subjects with stress-related disorders (PTSD, adjustment disorder, or other stress-related conditions) and a mean age of forty-one were followed for ten years and compared to 1,064,640 matched unexposed individuals as well as 126,652 full siblings.[14] The exposure to a clinical diagnosis of stress-related disorders was significantly associated with a 36 percent increased risk of autoimmune disease. That's huge, not just the implication that stress begets pathophysiological changes and potentially autoimmunity, but that *JAMA* was acknowledging a sea change in our understanding of how we might advance the way that we test for vulnerability and progression to autoimmunity.

It's not just *JAMA* asking us to look earlier in the process, upstream from the final diagnosis of an autoimmune disease. One of the imprints of the esteemed journal *Nature* published a similar finding in animals, demonstrating that immune changes occur in response to stress.[15] However, much of the literature in humans has been focused not on regular folks like you and me, but on people traumatized by miliary service and their subsequent development of autoimmune disease.[16]

In medicine, we call the gradient effect, the middle ground from health to disease, "preclinical autoimmune disease." It's a curious label, because it suggests that we are exploring a problem before doctors want to pay attention to it. Not this doctor.

In a newer publication titled "Preclinical Autoimmune Disease: A Comparison of Rheumatoid Arthritis, Systemic Lupus Erythematosus,

Multiple Sclerosis, and Type 1 Diabetes," researchers from the University of Amsterdam reviewed the gradient effect and how many diseases overlap in their development: "In general, we observed some notable similarities such as a North-South gradient of decreasing prevalence, a female preponderance (except for T1D), major genetic risk factors at the HLA level, partly overlapping cytokine profiles and lifestyle risk factors such as obesity, smoking, and stress. The latter risk factors are known to produce a state of chronic systemic low-grade inflammation."[17]

A key commonality of all four autoimmune diseases is that the average time patients experience no symptoms or minimal symptoms may last many years, "suggesting a gradually evolving interaction between the genetic profile and the environment. Part of the abnormalities may be present in unaffected family members, and autoimmune diseases can also cluster in families." An example is an increased level of high-sensitivity CRP, a marker of inflammation. The team found that it rises approximately five years prior to the onset of symptoms.[18] They end the review article on an upbeat note: "A promising strategy for prevention of autoimmune diseases might be to address adverse lifestyle factors by public health measures at the population level." Amen, that's the purpose of this book!

You might wonder what types of tests these journal articles assessed . . . of course, they all looked at the PINE network: measures of the stress response in the hypothalamic-pituitary-adrenal axis,[19] the autonomic nervous system,[20] and immune mediators[21]—the networks that we described in Part 1.[22] (See notes.[23])

All of this points to the fact that autoimmunity is not an on/off switch but a gradient from health to disease. You don't have a perfect immune system and hormones one day and then the next day they are a hot mess. So what do we do with this knowledge? We can look at function, not just track the changes in biomarkers.

That's where a functional approach can be a helpful paradigm. I've written about this topic for the past fifteen years: I was taught to look at disease only. For instance, with the stress hormone cortisol, you are either healthy ("normal" cortisol), or you have the extreme of nearly zero cortisol (a rare endocrinopathy called Addison's disease that's autoimmune in nature), or you have the other extreme of excessively, pathologically high cortisol (a slightly less rare endocrinopathy called Cushing's disease). There was no consideration of the function between the extreme states. We need to acknowledge that between these extremes, like so-called normal cortisol and adrenal insufficiency of Addison's, is a lot of suffering for individual patients. This gets dismissed wholesale by an approach that behaves as if health and disease are binary. When we consider the upstream and gradual loss of function, we open ourselves to a world of possibility where we might be able to intervene before things get worse and an autoimmune disease is diagnosed. Instead of the default approach that I learned on the conventional side of medicine—that these people who are suffering pre-disease are well and just have psychosomatic issues, and how about a referral to a psychiatrist or therapist—we can now acknowledge that we need to consider all of the many pathways that become dysfunctional years in advance of that autoimmune illness that are affecting not just the mind and psyche but the body as well. They are the walking wounded and need our help. Maybe you're one of them.

Initiation of Hormonal Flux

An initiation is an expansion of consciousness, a shift from one state of being to another. It can be biological or spiritual, and often both. While you may not consider pregnancy or the shortening cycle length of perimenopause in this way, I invite you to consider your own timeline and life transitions, and how they may be impacting the process of autoimmunity. The variety and steepness of hormonal transition in women may be part of the reason why we are more affected by autoimmunity— 70 to 80 percent of people with autoimmune disease are assigned female at birth, and 85 percent of people with multiple autoimmune diseases are women.[24]

Pregnancy may trigger an autoimmune disorder. It affects the onset and progression of autoimmune disease by modulating the chemicals that T cells, known as cytokines, make during gestation and postpartum. Antibodies that the mother produces may enter the fetal circulation and potentially cause harm, and this even has been shown to be associated with mental health issues later in offspring up to early adulthood, particularly for mothers with type 1 diabetes and rheumatoid arthritis.[25] Autoimmune conditions can have both positive and negative impacts, ranging from miscarriage to remission. One of the most common conditions that I see is autoimmune attack on the thyroid causing

---

A PUPPY'S NERVOUS SYSTEM BY JO ILFELD, PHD

Learning about how trauma affects the nervous system from Dr. Sara has made me much more aware about how I handle my newest puppy. I can see the nervous system development happening in my puppy every day, and instead of being frustrated about the barking and telling him to be quiet (definitely tempting!), I'm trying to help him learn ways to rebalance his own nervous system.

As a puppy, he's incredibly scared of new people coming into the house. I can see that once a repairman enters our house, even if they're not close to the puppy, he starts barking and barking (while our eleven-year-old dog barely looks up from her nap). The repairman entering his house feels overwhelming to the new puppy, and his system goes into high alert and he can't calm himself. Since I've realized his cortisol was spiking and he couldn't self-regulate, I've started to move his crate away from where he can see the repairman (such as in my or my husband's office). This way he has a familiar presence, and he can't see the offending person. This allows him to calm down. Similarly, on his first hike, I realized that the combination of a new environment and other dogs was too overwhelming, so we found a path with almost no one on it, and he was able to only deal with one stressor, being in a new place, without the overlapping stressors of new people and dogs to fear.

Having this puppy as my three kids are departing the nest has made me aware how crucial parents are to helping their kids regulate their nervous systems when they're young, before they can on their own. It makes me appreciate even more how working on regulating your nervous system as a guardian (of kids, animals, or anyone) pays it forward when you can help your dependents learn to lean on you as their nervous systems are developing.

---

inflammation and destruction of the thyroid gland, diagnosed in the postpartum period.

Perimenopause, the years that escort you from regular menstrual cycles to the one-year anniversary of no period, known as menopause, is associated with increased autoimmunity. Like the other massive endocrinological transitions, perimenopause creates significant changes on the immune system with regard to the interface of hormones and innate and adaptive immunity, leading to greater susceptibility to autoimmune disease. The effect is bidirectional, and a previous diagnosis of an autoimmune disease may impact the transition. Estrogen, progesterone, testosterone, oxytocin, prolactin, and leptin are known to modulate immune balance.[26] More toxic stress may be a tipping point that shifts a woman from immune balance to imbalance.[27]

As I've witnessed thousands of clients going through the chemically induced growth process of pregnancy, postpartum, perimenopause, and menopause, I see some people who navigate well and some who do not. Those who navigate well don't view their symptoms as nuisances to be medicated away as quickly as possible but rather as cues, messages from the body and mind, to be explored, decoded, and addressed. They may also, but not always, seek to use information and guidance from expanded states of reality to gain insight and direction. They acknowledge and commit to healing their trauma and to responding differently to the inevitable stressors of a busy, full life. They are willing to be self-reflective, without harsh judgment, and to grow past old limits.

Back to Aaron and Irritable Bowel Syndrome

Aaron had seen other doctors before me for his scalp. He was given topical steroids to apply to the psoriatic plaques. What are steroids? A derivative of stress hormones. The body becomes adjusted to the high levels of stress hormones from trauma, and sometimes needs the high dose of stress hormones to calm down. That's true not just for psoriasis, but for most autoimmune conditions we treat with oral steroids, from inflammatory bowel disease to lupus to rheumatoid arthritis. While treating symptoms with steroids is considered a risk/benefit decision, as an integrative physician, I encourage my patients to consider addressing the root cause, which can often be traced back to trauma and how it originally disrupted the stress response system.

Studies have associated psychological distress, trauma, and immune activation to bowel disorders, such as IBS and gastroesophageal reflux disease (indigestion). These bowel disorders are linked to the tendency to develop allergies (atopy) and certain autoimmune diseases.[28] Research has also shown that adverse experiences in childhood, a way of measuring trauma, are more common in people with IBS compared to controls,[29] and people with IBS have a higher rate of fear and dissociation associated with early adverse life events.[30] While women in the original studies of adverse childhood experiences (ACEs) report a higher rate of trauma, there is no sex difference in the link between ACE score and

IBS. Fortunately, protective factors, such as confiding in others, can decrease the chance of IBS.[31]

Even if your doctor is not yet aware that IBS is sometimes considered an autoimmune disease, the symptoms can mimic other autoimmune conditions such as celiac disease, Crohn's disease, and ulcerative colitis, and researchers have found a link between exhausted immune cells and IBS.[32] Further, many of the conditions that we consider in this book—such as autoimmune diseases, anxiety, and depression—are connected to the gut-brain axis, a messed-up state of balance, and changes in gut microbes that result from upstream problems related to stress and the stress chemicals, including CRH, the molecule that makes you release cortisol and also pokes holes in your gut lining.[33]

Evidence continues to mount regarding stressful life events and health risk, but we still have misunderstandings and weaknesses in the scientific literature worth mentioning. The largest study that we have of trauma is the adverse childhood experiences (ACE) survey performed in the 1990s. The Centers for Disease Control and Prevention, in partnership with Kaiser Permanente, created a list of childhood traumas that were the top ten most common among the initial subjects in the San Diego study. The ten most common became the "ACE score." However, the ACE score misses many stressful life events, such as violence outside of the home, poverty, racism and other forms of discrimination, being born premature, bullying, observing a sibling getting abused, losing a caregiver, or being in foster care or the juvenile justice system. It also misses protective factors, like supportive relationships and community services, and individual factors, like grit and resilience. Yet the score still provides the most robust data we have showing a direct link between ACEs and disease in middle age, and not just mental health problems.

Trauma Leads to Heightened Sensitivity

When I asked Aaron what he was like as a child, he described that he had been highly sensitive for as long as he could remember. He wasn't sure if he was born exquisitely sensitive to his environment—to sound, tone of voice, loud noises, cigarette smoke, perfumes, judgment—or if that developed in response to stress. Maybe his intrauterine experience knitted into his chromosomes an exaggerated stress response, as he listened to his father rage against his older siblings or his mother. Perhaps the trauma was passed on like soul wounds by ancestors, including grandparents who fled a genocide (you'll learn more on intergenerational trauma in chapter 3). It's a classic case of the chicken-and-egg conundrum, of determining cause and effect. Sometimes you don't know the precise and singular cause—you are just left with the effects.

Sensitivity to environment is the hallmark of a child with trauma. The more sensitive a child is, the more the child feels the stress and pain of the environment in which they are raised. That feels bidirectional to me—that a sensitive child feels the stress and pain acutely in their environment, and that a stressful environment may make a vulnerable child more sensitive. This observation was described by Alice Miller, MD, a Swiss/German and Jewish psychoanalyst who wrote in 1979 *The Drama of the Gifted Child*.[34] She documented how sensitive and alert children learn at an early age to adapt to others' needs and to repress rather than to acknowledge and integrate intense feelings because they may not be accepted by the parents. Sensitive kids may then flee their repressed pain with achievement, alcohol, or drugs, among other things. Those children who seek achievement to cover their pain are often recognized as gifted, though of course not all gifted kids have a history of trauma.

We all differ in how strongly we respond to similar experiences, and the difference becomes more marked in response to negative ones. Environmental sensitivity is defined as the ability to register and process external stimuli,[35] and when you look around at your own family of origin, you will probably notice that people with low sensitivity tend to coexist with people with high sensitivity. Less than half of environmental sensitivity is genetic.[36]

When I was parenting my kids, we called highly sensitive children like Aaron "spirited"—that is, more intense, sensitive, persistent, perceptive, and resistant to change than the average.[37] Fifteen years later, Michael Pluess and his group at Queen Mary University in London offered the latest approach to assessing environmental sensitivity among children and why one sibling can differ so much from another. He classifies differences in sensitivity into three groups—low, medium, and high.[38] Think of it this way: the orchid is the most sensitive to environment, the dandelion is the most hearty and resilient, and the tulip is somewhere in between.[39]

The majority of my patients with autoimmune diseases are orchids, a few are tulips, and almost none are dandelions.

Measuring Aaron

In my consultation with Aaron, we found the following hallmarks of autoimmune disease, all of which we will explore more fully in the chapters to come.

- Loss of gut boundaries: low stomach acid, low secretory immunoglobulin, and abnormalities of the gut microbiome. In Aaron's stool, certain bacteria, like prevotella,[40] dominated, which can trigger the autoimmune pathway in the body.
- Increased intestinal permeability (leaky gut), which can be linked to leaky brain (loss of the blood-brain barrier integrity), which can cause inflammation in the brain and brain fog.
- Hormone imbalances: low cortisol, typical in trauma survivors, and low DHEA. Both low cortisol and low DHEA are common in people with autoimmune disease.

Aaron's gut, microbiome, and hormones were out of whack, leading to an immune system imbalance, which can further lead to uncontrolled and widespread inflammation. However, not all people with a history of trauma have results like Aaron's. A study of thirty-five women with autoimmune disease showed they had excessively high cortisol levels (as measured in their hair), and when you look at a graph of cortisol levels over the day, total cortisol load is higher as measured by the area under the curve.[41] In other words, the control system for hormones gets wonky in both the short and long term, leading to abnormal cortisol levels that can be high or low or a combination of the two (e.g., low in the morning, high at night).

I notice while talking to Aaron that he would space out on occasion. He'd stare at his phone while I was asking difficult questions about his emotional life. Aaron has alexithymia, a personality trait characterized by difficulty recognizing, differentiating, and verbalizing feelings. You can think of alexithymia as a form of emotional blindness, experienced by about one in ten people. It's as if the lexicon for describing feelings is lacking. Alexithymia is associated with several autoimmune conditions affecting the skin, including psoriasis, vitiligo, alopecia areata, and chronic hives.[42] Alexithymia and psoriasis are particularly closely linked.[43] Other autoimmune conditions have shown a connection too, including Hashimoto's thyroiditis,[44] rheumatoid arthritis,[45] and Ménière's disease (a condition in which the immune response attacks the inner ear and may cause vertigo).[46]

One study from the University of Rome of fifty patients with rheumatoid arthritis and fifty-one patients with psoriasis showed that 38.6 percent had alexithymia, 26.7 percent were borderline, and 34.7 percent did not have alexithymia. Think of alexithymia as another piece of the puzzle that shows us how trauma gets under the skin and creates dysregulation. One study of 306 people with autoimmune disease suggested a relationship between childhood trauma and autoimmune disorders, which was mediated by dissociation and alexithymia compared to healthy controls.[47] Unfortunately, even though research shows a strong connection between trauma, dissociation, alexithymia, and autoimmune disorders, not enough clinicians are making the connections—for example, by asking about trauma or looking for signs of dissociation or alexithymia—in the treatment of autoimmunity.

Wrap-Up

While the immediate pain of trauma is important to consider, it's the long-term health consequences that are the subject of this book—and importantly, the journey into expanded states of consciousness that may allow you to transcend old hurts so that you can create a life of healing and balance, from your hormones to your immune cells to your soul. In my experience, I observe patients who can leverage consciousness to call off the attack on their own tissues and reduce autoimmune activity. Science is slow to confirm, but science tends to confirm what the body already knows.

We are finally aware of the full gamut of mental health issues that may occur after trauma exposure, but we are new to the physical health issues that may occur as a result of trauma. As Gabor Maté has written, trauma causes distortions in how we interpret the world and how we are situated in it. Health issues, relationships, and behavior can be problematic. Chronic conditions may not resolve, particularly those with a stress component like IBS and other autoimmune diseases. In his book *In the Realm of Hungry Ghosts*, Dr. Maté states the following: "Unwittingly, we write the story of our future from narratives based on the past. . . . Mindful awareness can bring into consciousness those hidden, past-based perspectives so that they no longer frame our worldview. Choice begins the moment you disidentify from the mind and its conditioned patterns, the moment you become present. . . . Until you reach that point, you are unconscious."[48] It is my opinion after thirty years of medical practice that your level of consciousness and presence may impact your risk of disease, including autoimmunity. We'll delve deeper into the origins and measurement of your trauma in the next chapter.

CHAPTER 3

Understanding Autoimmunity Triggered by Trauma

In trauma recovery, we want to feel safe enough to feel activated and to know that's not going to mean something bad is happening. We want to develop our ability to let go of defensive states so that we can receive the care we need. We want to soften without collapsing, relax without shutting down, and settle into stillness without feeling stuck.

—ARIELLE SCHWARTZ, PHD[1]

In her midfifties, my patient Tamara was diagnosed with type 1 diabetes, an autoimmune disease that attacks the islet cells that produce insulin in the pancreas. As Tamara explained when I took her history, she hit perimenopause at age forty-seven, which brought monthly menstrual migraines that prescriptions didn't fix. On her own, she discovered that a daily organic green drink resolved them, but ultimately the greens did not help her increasing blood lipids, particularly triglycerides. At age fifty-two, Tamara had night sweats and hot flashes, belly fat, swelling, and sleep issues. By age fifty-five, she gave up her beloved green drink because she wondered if it was spiking her triglycerides. After a few weeks off the greens, Tamara felt off: brain fog, dizziness, light-headedness, ringing in her ears, moodiness, and weirdly, weight loss. Blood work showed a high fasting glucose of 110 mg/dL that no doctor mentioned to her at the time. Eventually, she was diagnosed with late-onset type 1 diabetes with an A1C of ten. Tamara's endocrinologist explained the cause of type 1 diabetes was irrelevant and undiscoverable and that she needed to start "lifetime insulin use" because research showed limited pancreas function would be preserved by insulin therapy. She politely declined, requesting less drastic treatment. Tamara was told to lose twenty pounds, take metformin, and watch her diet. No one asked her about trauma.

In our appointments, we explored the root cause of her autoimmune attack on her pancreas. After discussing the potential trigger of trauma, Tamara said, "My resilience keeps me from recognizing all the little traumas in my life added up to one big Trauma at some point. I notice significant spikes in my glucose when I have periods of high stress. For instance, most of the time it is very steady now, but when my son had a near-fatal accident a few weeks ago, the cortisol/adrenaline rush was something. I can now recognize and pinpoint that as a 'super stress' event, and when looking back, I would have those regularly with both parental and spousal conflicts. I have no doubt that suffering the little traumas and their associated glucose increase overloaded my system and contributed to my development of an autoimmune condition."

Connecting Trauma and Autoimmunity: Trauma Breaks the Container

In the quest to understand how trauma may be linked to autoimmunity, we can look at both childhood and adult trauma, and consider the healthy versus less healthy response to trauma exposure. As Tamara's case illustrates, adversity—emotional, physical, environmental—impacts the development of cells, tissues, organs, and physiology, especially the delicate balance of homeostasis.

When adversity occurs in childhood, the impacts are not only more pronounced but also longer lasting. Children are not small adults; when they experience, for example, disruption in healthy parenting and a lack of protection, they are more vulnerable than adults to developing inappropriate cellular processes and subsequent dysfunction of bodily systems. Damage seems to affect primarily the gut, brain, immune, and endocrine systems, but the fallout is much broader. Nearly all systems that have been studied show dysfunction after significant childhood trauma, including the gut-brain axis, microbiome, and gut-liver-bile acid axis. While the damage affects development and homeostasis of these tissues, organs, and systems, the damage is also associated with later-life conditions, including autoimmune disease, the primordial link between trauma and autoimmunity. You might think that disrupted programming is rare, but the truth is that it's far more common than you may realize. I suspect the same is true of trauma in adulthood, depending on the level of trauma and the person's resourcing, or the capacity to identify and utilize coping skills to help deal with difficult reactions. Resources help us to keep calm and in the present moment.

Trauma—especially childhood or developmental trauma—breaks the sacred container of care and protection that our body's physiology is designed to provide for us to thrive. Think of the sacred container as your experience of safety in your body. Without it, we lose a sense of choice, control, and containment in our lives. That particular loss ultimately leads one to feel overwhelmed and set off by ordinary events, like a difficult conversation, which perpetuates the threat response.

It's not that you can't heal trauma that occurred when you were young; we just need to know what we are working with and how to repair it in order to re-create wholeness and access effective resources and regulation. We need to know the original shaping of the person—the injury and how it may have led to dysregulation. We also want to assess the ongoing social and behavioral experiences, and we need to learn how to work with the emotional loops that we can get caught in, the ones that are no longer useful—such as negative self-talk and beliefs and behaviors—and that could be driving autoimmunity.

As we dive deeper into the specifics of wounding that trauma causes in the body, allow me to remind you that not everyone with autoimmune disease has experienced trauma, and not everyone with trauma develops autoimmune disease. Further, not everyone with autoimmune disease needs to resolve trauma in order to heal autoimmunity. Rather, autoimmunity and trauma are sometimes coexistent, and for some people, both need to be addressed for the greatest healing.

Tamara developed an autoimmune disease in perimenopause. She has leaky gut and signs of an incomplete stress response and resolution, including abnormal cortisol levels.

Sabine, also a survivor of significant childhood trauma, has not developed autoimmune disease. She is learning how her body can have a healthier response to trauma.

Sabine is a forty-four-year-old chief executive officer of a technology company. She lives with a high ACE score of thirteen (see the ACE questionnaire later in this chapter, on page 48). As Sabine describes it, she is full of rage and spends thousands of dollars on therapy. Someone tried to mug her last month and the perpetrator ran away, scared. "I'm like, pick a non-angry woman, you MF. I'll beat your ass." She felt like a bad-ass bitch in the moment, but it took her five hours to stop shaking—an example of mobilization and action.

That's Sabine's trauma talking and healing. It shows up in different ways, and shaking is an example of mobilization and action that can return us to homeostasis, or balance.

Trauma as Unresolved Stress Response

You are now becoming familiar with how trauma interacts with the body. External triggers, especially from but not limited to childhood, may or may not be handled in the way that our bodies were designed to function. Now let's get into the details of what trauma does to the body—how it can restrict the mental, emotional, and physical capacity of a person. At its simplest, you can think of trauma as an unresolved stress response.

Let's start with the healthy stress response to an acute event that your body was designed to resolve. You experience a trauma, like learning from the doctor that your loved one is seriously ill. After the trauma exposure, you feel the flush of increasing cortisol, the main stress hormones. You leave the doctor's office with your loved one and go on a walk, mobilizing big muscle groups in your legs and discharging the stress that you both feel as you talk through the details of what just happened. You notice a sense of resolution, a return to homeostasis. *Importantly, there is nothing wrong with you, an individual who experiences a trauma.* You are a person responding to something that was wrong in the environment—in this case, deeply distressing news about someone you love. Peter Levine, PhD, is a psychotherapist who developed a body-awareness approach to healing trauma called somatic experiencing. He describes the normal stress response in wild animals similarly: they encounter a threat, deal with it, then recover from stress via tremoring spasms of their body to complete the fight-or-flight process.

In contrast, there is the less healthy or more trauma-conditioned stress response that may lead to the sensation of ongoing threat, long after the trauma exposure. The first two steps are the same: trauma exposure to a stressful event and increased cortisol. Instead of mobilization and action, there is incomplete mobilization, sometimes a freeze response, associated with high arousal. Imagine, in the previous scenario of the bad news from the doctor, that you froze when you heard the details. You and your loved one drove home in silence, drank a few glasses of wine, and watched television. You didn't process the experience together. You couldn't sleep that night because you were on high alert. You haven't had a good night's sleep since that day and cannot get the situation out of your mind. You avoid the subject. The trauma-related stress is unresolved.

Sometimes it can be incomplete mobilization into helplessness with a collapse or faint response, associated with low arousal. The body does not experience resolution, and it feels like the threat is ongoing. Most people don't feel it as incomplete resolution; rather, they feel like they are struggling most of the time, embattled, shut down, often lashing out in relationships. The implications range from macro to micro—high-conflict marriages, difficulty staying employed and getting along with colleagues, estranged children plus blood sugar abnormalities, fainting episodes, rising calcium deposits in their arteries, gut issues. They want things to be different, and they may recall as children investing energetically in a wish to be somewhere different, to be someone different—this was my rallying cry as a kid—but even though it may be a common sentiment for a child, it can sometimes be lacerating to the psyche, to the sense of wholeness. Over time, it becomes exhausting.

Thoughts become our biology. Your thoughts change your cells and how they function. Consider a thought to be an electromagnetic field and neuroendocrine signal that can be positive or negative. Thoughts cause our body's biochemistry to shift.[2] For example, we take that incomplete resolution and start to shut down the full range of authentic feelings. Maybe we then try to control the environment to create more harmony, though that rarely works.

That's also trauma talking. It shows up in different ways. Some of us fight and shake from the massive surge of stress hormones, like a wild gazelle or Sabine. Some of us freeze and dissociate. Sabine continues: "Having so much consistent trauma, as a way of life, means recognizing and finding a baseline for normalcy is really tricky." Absolutely true: in this chapter we will cover the origins of trauma and how that can be measured in the PINE system, using questionnaires.

Russian author Leo Tolstoy famously wrote that "all happy families are alike, but every unhappy family is unhappy in its own way."[3] Trauma is similar. Those of us who have experienced trauma—and that's nearly all of us—are traumatized uniquely. Some of us endure potentially toxic stress and remain healthy. Others feel overwhelmed by an experience or multiple experiences over time, and develop soul wounds. (I define "soul" as the spiritual, nonphysical quality of a person or animal.)

Even with the same exposure, some people experience full resolution and homeostasis, some experience PTSD, and some experience complex PTSD that includes problems with interpersonal dynamics, negative self-concept, and how the person expresses emotion (known as affect). While some trauma survivors fit the stereotype of a war veteran with flashbacks, nightmares, and moral injury, we need to recognize that some of us have

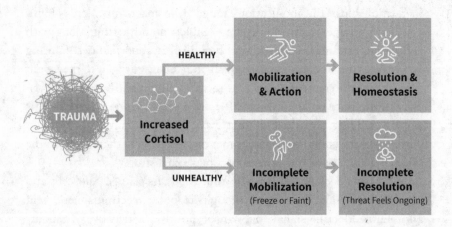

more subtle situations of partial PTSD (also known as subthreshold PTSD). These folks don't meet all the criteria, but the micro to macro issues of trauma are still operating behind the scenes, dismantling bodily barriers that lead to an immune system out of balance and may overactivate into autoimmunity. Gabor Maté, MD, wrote that trauma is not what happened to us but is the ongoing dysregulation that still exists in the body. One path of the dysregulation can be autoimmunity.

Since autoimmunity so often originates in trauma, it is important for you to dig deeper and understand whether you have enough to change your health trajectory.

Trauma Is Prevalent

People with trauma—Radha in the introduction, Kristina in chapter 1, Aaron in chapter 2—are not alone. Indeed, studies of childhood trauma show that more people experience serious trauma than not—approximately 64 percent of us, even employed, mostly white, middle-class, college-educated people with health insurance.[4]

However, just because trauma is prevalent doesn't make it normal or healthy. It could be an overwhelming experience from childhood, like divorce or neglect, as Aaron experienced, or even surviving the fear, uncertainty, and losses of the recent pandemic. We can now measure trauma before birth, known as intergenerational trauma. That could be a past genocide that affected your ancestors, or a mother who was pregnant during the September 11 terrorist attacks and passed on a greater risk of autoimmunity to her fetus. One of my colleagues was pregnant and living near the Pentagon on September 11. Her daughter, now in her early twenties, struggles with inflammatory bowel disease and Rayaud's. Trauma has affected nearly all of us.

While Aaron's appraisal of his childhood experiences did not seem to merit mention, science disagrees. The more traumatic your childhood, the higher the ACE score, and the greater your risk of future health conditions of all types. Similar to other toxic exposures from the environment, such as to arsenic or phthalates, ACEs can harm a child's developing brain, gut, endocrine, and immune system, provoking a change in how the child responds to stress and damaging the immune system in ways that may not show up until decades later.

The original study of ACEs was performed at Kaiser Permanente, a health maintenance organization in San Diego, and measured childhood trauma and stressors in middle-class people who were employed. From the seventeen thousand study subjects, we know an ACE score of four or higher increases Aaron's (or anyone with a similar ACE score) risk of depression by 460 percent and suicide by 1,200 percent compared to a person with an ACE score of zero.[5] He's also more likely to have autoimmune disease, which is when the immune system becomes confused and attacks parts of the body that it's supposed to shield. Specifically, patients with psoriasis[6] and IBS experience more ACEs,[7] though the ACE/IBS connection may be stronger in females.[8] While we've known about the link between ACEs and IBS for nearly thirty years,[9] more research is needed to help us understand the precise mechanisms behind the link.

WHAT'S YOUR ADVERSE CHILDHOOD EXPERIENCES (ACE) SCORE?

Before your eighteenth birthday . . .

1. Did a parent or other adult in the household often or very often swear at you, insult you, put you down, or humiliate you?

2. Did a parent or other adult in the household often or very often act in a way that made you afraid that you might be physically hurt?

3. Did a parent or other adult in the household often or very often push, grab, slap, or throw something at you?

4. Did a parent or other adult in the household often or very often hit you so hard that you had marks or were injured?

5. Did an adult or person at least five years older than you ever touch or fondle you or have you touch their body in a sexual way?

6. Did an adult or person at least five years older than you ever attempt or actually have oral, anal, or vaginal intercourse with you?

7. Did you often or very often feel that no one in your family loved you or thought you were important or special?

8. Did you often or very often feel that your family didn't look out for one another, feel close to one another, or support one another?

9. Did you often or very often feel that you didn't have enough to eat, had to wear dirty clothes, and had no one to protect you?

10. Did you often or very often feel that our parents were too drunk or high to take care of you or take you to the doctor if you needed it?

Triggering Autoimmunity

Now that we've covered the normal and abnormal stress response, we can connect the dots to the gut and immune system, and begin to see how an abnormal stress response may set up a person for autoimmune disease and disorder. Understanding the link between trauma and auto-immunity can help point us in the direction of how to heal from it.

While there are about one hundred known autoimmune diseases, research indicates that the proximate triad of autoimmunity is a combi-nation of genetic predisposition, increased intestinal permeability (i.e., loss of the integrity of the intestinal lining that allows things to pass through to the person's bloodstream that don't belong, like bacteria and other inflammatory pathogens—also known as leaky gut), and a trigger that turns on the genes.

11. Were your parents ever separated or divorced?

12. Was your mother or stepmother sometimes, often, or very often pushed, grabbed, or slapped or had something thrown at her?

13. Was your mother or stepmother sometimes, often, or very often kicked, bitten, hit with a fist, or hit with something hard?

14. Was your mother or stepmother sometimes, often, or very often repeatedly hit over at least a few minutes or threatened with a gun or knife?

15. Did you live with anyone who was a problem drinker or alcoholic or who used street drugs?

16. Was a household member depressed or mentally ill, or did a household member attempt suicide?

17. Did a household member go to prison?

*Note: The ACE questionnaires are not copyrighted, and there are no fees for their use. Some forms of the ACE questionnaire combine questions or add additional questions.

Interpretation: A score of zero means that you had minimal exposure to trauma, at least as measured by the original questionnaire. However, most of us have a score of one or higher. A score of four or higher occurs in one in six adults in the United States. If your score is one or higher, or you know someone with a score of one or higher, that's a positive childhood trauma history. Read on.

Other factors that add to the triggering and predispose people to autoimmunity include the following:

- **INFLAMMATION**, whether it's from an unhealthy diet, poor sleep, high stress, toxin overload, or infection.
- **FEMALE SEX.** Women are well-known to mount a stronger immune system response to infection and vaccines—and that stronger immune system can backfire, leading to a woman's greater risk of autoimmunity.
- **HORMONE IMBALANCE.** Ever wondered why puberty, pregnancy, postpartum, perimenopause, and menopause can be a trigger for autoimmunity? It's the hormones, particularly the interplay of estrogen and progesterone.
- **INFECTION.** Specific infections have been linked to autoimmunity, including the connection between autoimmune thyroid disease (both Hashimoto's and

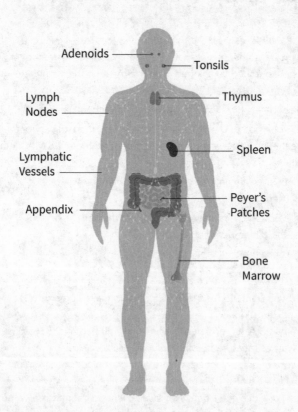

MEET YOUR IMMUNE SYSTEM

The immune system is like a private security detail that protects you from invaders. It consists of a complex network of cells, tissues, organs, and signaling molecules that help the body fight infection and other diseases. While it can seem mysterious, I'd like to break it down for you so that you become intimate with it, which is the first step in healing. The immune security system has three main jobs:

- Fight disease-causing germs like viruses, bacteria, parasites, and fungi and remove them from the body
- Recognize and, if possible, neutralize environmental harms, like chemicals, including silicone implants
- Track adverse changes in the body, like the growth of cancer cells

The main structures of the immune system that fight infection and attempt to keep you safe consist of the following:

- **TONSILS** and **ADENOIDS**. Tonsils are the first line of defense against germs that you eat or inhale, like the common cold virus, and are located in the back of the throat. Adenoids are a collection of tissue high in the throat, behind the nose. Tonsils and adenoids work by trapping germs coming in via the mouth and nose.
- **LYMPHATIC SYSTEM** includes the tubes known as lymphatic vessels and clusters known as lymph nodes. Note that "lymph" and "lymphoid" refer to tissue responsible for producing a type of blood cell known as a lymphocyte, which centers in lymph nodes and organs plus is dispersed throughout the body.
- **THYMUS** is the primary "lymphoid" organ of the immune system, which makes and develops immune cells called thymus cell lymphocytes, known as T cells. It is located in the upper front part of the chest behind the sternum or chest bone. It shrinks starting in your teen years in both size and function.
- **SPLEEN** is another organ in the immune system, and it's like a large lymph node that filters blood.
- **PEYER'S PATCHES** are clusters of cells in your intestine, especially the part of the small intestine known as the ileum.
- **APPENDIX.** We used to think that the appendix was a vestigial or unnecessary organ, but now we know it's a lymphoid organ that assists with the development of B lymphocytes, another type of white blood cell, and their production of a type of antibody called immunoglobulin A.

- **BONE MARROW** is the spongy tissue inside large bones that makes blood cells, including white blood cells, red blood cells, and platelets. When you peek inside the marrow, you find young and immature cells called stem cells.

Cells in these structures set a perimeter and shield you from troublesome invaders, not just bacteria and viruses but also cancer cells.

The cast of characters or cells in the immune network is lengthy, ranging from white blood cells to monocytes, macrophages, and mast cells, among others. The places they accumulate—including the bone marrow, thymus, spleen, lymph nodes, tonsils, and lymphatic vessels—are equally varied. Many immune cells create tools to vanquish invaders, like antibodies (proteins) and cytokines (chemical messengers that can affect other cells, such as interferon, interleukin, and growth factors). Other cells known as macrophages surround and kill bugs, remove dead cells, and trigger the activation of other immune system cells.

Humans have three types of immunity: innate, adaptive, and passive. Innate is the general immune protection you have at birth—such as your skin, which is a barrier that blocks germs from entering the body. Adaptive immunity develops as you age, such as when you are exposed to an infection or receive a vaccine. Passive immunity comes from another source; for example, the antibodies in a woman's breast milk provide a baby with temporary protection to diseases she has been exposed to.

This miraculous system that keeps us healthy despite constant challenges is not foolproof. Indeed, the immune system can get befuddled, leading it to attack the healthy tissues that it's supposed to shield. That's autoimmunity.

Men and women have the same immune cells, tools, and pathways to protect against disease, but hormones can modify the activity—for example, estrogen and progesterone can make women respond more strongly to vaccination. Generally, women have greater innate and adaptive immune response compared to men, which leads to quicker clearance of germs but can backfire and lead to a greater risk of autoimmune and other inflammatory conditions.[10]

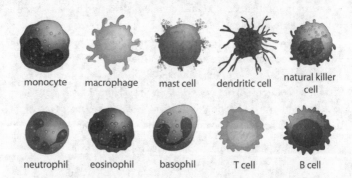

monocyte   macrophage   mast cell   dendritic cell   natural killer cell

neutrophil   eosinophil   basophil   T cell   B cell

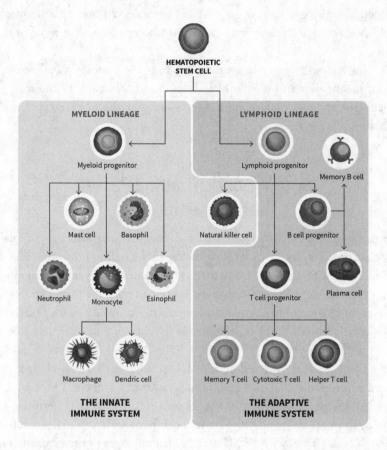

Graves' disease) and *Yersinia enterocolitica*, bacteria found in contaminated water and food.[11] Immune thrombocytopenic purpura, an autoimmune disease where the body creates autoantibodies against proteins on the platelets, is associated with human immunodeficiency virus (HIV), hepatitis C virus, and *Helicobacter pylori*. Sometimes you can have an infection and it takes years for autoimmune disease to develop or be diagnosed.

For these factors to activate the immune system, they behave as a trigger that turns on the genetic predisposition. The trigger can be understood as the root cause, such as factory food, hormonal shifts, toxic stress, toxic culture, racism, misogyny, or . . . trauma. Then the triad of genetics, leaky gut, and trigger collide to cause chronic inflammation, which then causes the immune system to be reactive all or most of the time.

The triad turns on the immune system to the "autoimmune" setting. That means we can potentially address modifiable parts of the triad— leaky gut and the underlying triggers—to reset the immune system to health.

Soul Wounds: Trauma Passed Transgenerationally

You inherit DNA from your parents, and you can also inherit their gene expression, like a sticky note on the DNA telling it how to behave, a note that can be passed down through families. Parents and grandparents who experience a traumatic event can pass the gene expression down to their children and grandchildren, according to the research of Rachel Yehuda, PhD, a professor of psychiatry and neurosciences at Mount Sinai hospital.

Think of that sticky note like a soul wound that can change the type of molecule that the gene is programmed to make. Dr. Yehuda's work, looking at survivors of the Holocaust and the 9/11 terrorist attacks, shows that the effect of trauma can be inherited. First, she found that 9/11 survivors with PTSD actually had changes in the expression of the genes involved in stress response (such as FKBP5), and the immune system (such as major histocompatibility complex Class II).[12] Second, she found that mothers who were pregnant and directly exposed to the World Trade Center towers in the 9/11 terrorist attack and who subsequently developed post-traumatic stress disorder had a change in their levels of stress hormones—they had lower cortisol in the morning and evening, and the babies of 9/11-exposed mothers with PTSD had lower cortisol too.[13] In other words, when exposed to severe trauma, your DNA stays the same, but what it tells your body to do can change, and that instruction can get passed on to the next generation. This change in instructions can show up as behaviors that in turn can alter relationships, bonding, and beyond. Mothers with PTSD report their babies had higher infant distress, particularly caused by loud noises, new foods, and unfamiliar people.[14]

Wrap-Up

When you are exposed to trauma and aren't able to resolve it, you can lose coherence between body and mind. If you have the genetic vulnerability, increased gut permeability, and then a trigger, like trauma, you may be set up for autoimmunity.

Breakdown of fundamental coherence, a basic part of who you are and how you perceive the world, can lead to fragmentation and dissociation. In my opinion, this is the fundamental experience of trauma—loss of coherence. It can affect your sense of ease, safety, secure connection, and balance.

In the two cases shared earlier in this chapter, Tamara and Sabine, I am careful not to make sweeping comparisons. What's curious to me is that Sabine was in the throes of a trauma exposure—a mugging—and while she was afraid and angry, she suddenly realized she had a choice. She had agency, and she used it to mobilize against her assailant and protect herself. That's profound. While I cannot say that her immune system is following suit, so far she has avoided autoimmune illness.

You might ask, why are traumatic memories so sticky? How is the incomplete mobilization and resolution a setup for memories that feel like a real, ongoing threat? Why are some people vulnerable and others aren't? That's what we'll get into next.

If you are freaking out about a traumatic memory, please don't despair. This book is about how to reprogram the way that our cells, tissues, organs, and systems might have maladapted to trauma. I will help you with the shift, and we will take it one step at a time, starting with the body.

CHAPTER 4

Trauma Is Different for Men and Women

Lifetime trauma exposure is the norm in most countries.

—WORLD HEALTH ORGANIZATION[1]

M en and women respond differently to trauma. If we are to heal from trauma and autoimmunity, it's critical to understand the different responses without pitting one against the other, one up, one down, as if trauma were a zero-sum game. How might we resolve trauma together without blame or diminishing any person's experience? The more we know about the spectrum of profiles, male to female, the more we can then learn what works best for each of us—and all of us.[2]

We've covered in previous chapters how trauma gets embedded in your body as a break in the sacred container—a constriction on normal physiological regulation and mental health—and how trauma, big *T* or little *t*, can limit our ability to respond with full presence and authenticity. Many of us cope with a host of responses, including attachment wounding, a chronic freeze state of dissociation, or even, in my case, with intellectualization. (I feel safest when I fully understand what is happening and have always strived for knowledge to create safety, usually while also ignoring my body or disembodying.)

For a long time, doctors mistakenly assumed that what happens to men happens to all of us. Not necessarily so. Looking underneath the trauma response, I got curious about how those of us born male or female might respond differently, perhaps due to biology or societal influences. Understanding the sex and gender differences in how we experience trauma helps identify the most effective type of care for each of us in the resolution of trauma. In this chapter, we'll explore the reasons why sex and gender lead to a different response and can inform sex- and gender-based approaches that may be more effective than current psychological strategies. Answering these questions, however, presents its own hurdles due not only to complex sociophysiological interactions but also to the challenge of even defining sex and gender.

Sex Matters

Sex and gender are both determinants of health, but they are not the same, even though many researchers continue to conflate them. Gender is shaped by an individual's self-perception and identification plus societal constructs. Whereas sex at birth is binary and defined by your chromosomes (though there are cases of intersex), gender breaks the binary and is recognized as more fluid. Still, sex and gender have some relation to each other. For example, people born with male genital organs tend to have more muscle mass, longer limbs, stronger bones, and higher aerobic capacity.[3] People born with female genital organs tend to fatigue their muscles less, recover faster during endurance events, have higher body fat, and live longer. Our hormone levels also are different.[4] While there's a small gap in terms of sports performance, that gap closes to approximately 7 percent in Ironman-distance triathlons.[5] Go, women!

In this chapter, I will be using the terms of sex (female and male) and gender (women/women-identified and men/men-identified) intentionally to more accurately portray the underlying biological and sociocultural factors in play. This distinction will also help more fully capture the lived experiences of being born into different bodies. Even so, this language does not capture the full realm of possible sex and gender experiences—for example, some people, as mentioned, have middle-sex genitalia or consider themselves asexual or pansexual, some identify as nonbinary in gender, and more. We are a rich, beautiful species, after all! But even with this care, the challenges of understanding gender and sex differences with regard to trauma and autoimmunity go further, to the origin itself of what we know and how we know it.

Most Research Is Performed in Men

A quantitative review of twenty-five years of research, including 290 studies, showed that more than six in ten men experience potentially traumatic events versus five in ten women.[6] However, females make up only 2 percent of psychobiological research, mostly in rats.[7] In a new analysis published by the University of California at San Francisco, researchers found that when you look at the editors of academic journals in psychology and neuroscience—arguably one of the most powerful decision-making roles regarding the type of research that gets published—only 2 percent had a similar proportion of male and female editors and the rest of the journals had editors that were mostly male.[8] Both research and the deciders about research lack gender representation. No wonder we know so little about how to deal with sex differences in trauma. Yet even with the paucity of females included in studies, the sex differences are evident.

Most early research on trauma and PTSD was derived from studies of male veterans, particularly from the Vietnam War, which not only largely excluded women but also failed to capture men's full experience of trauma (beyond war). It wasn't until we began to study the effects of sexual assault that we finally developed a more complete understanding. Women who have experienced sexual assault react similarly to men in combat; both men and women report the symptoms of PTSD: hyperarousal, reexperiencing, avoidance, and numbing. Women and men experience the dissociative subtype of PTSD at equal rates.[9]

Beyond this set of responses, differences begin to emerge; for example, men experience less negative feelings about themselves such as shame compared to women. Frequently, symptoms are more common for women: more emotionality, somatic symptoms, anxiety and depression, defensive and palliative coping, and reexperiencing and anxious arousal, where you might feel a high level of vigilance.[10]

The higher rates of nearly all forms of autoimmune disease among women are one clue that potentially sex- and gender-based discrepancies in relation to trauma exist. Nevertheless, men develop autoimmune disease too, especially celiac, Addison's disease, autoimmune vasculitis, multiple sclerosis, lupus, inflammatory bowel disease, rheumatoid arthritis, and type 1 diabetes. In fact, type 1 diabetes affects men and women equally, and ankylosing spondylitis, associated with inflammatory arthritis of the spine and large joints, affects men slightly more than women. So we need to take a more refined look at what is operating beneath the hood that may represent a sex difference, in case a sex-based approach to treatment might be needed for the greatest healing.

We find, compared to men, women experience different types of toxic stress, and more of it, and more post-traumatic stress disorder (PTSD) than men, even with similar trauma exposure.

Gender Differences in Trauma Exposure and Response

Men and women's reaction to trauma is also different. In general, men become more aggressive whereas women tend to internalize the trauma more, leading to higher rates of anxiety, depression, and insomnia. Rates of PTSD are more than double in women compared to men (10 to 12 percent in women and 4 to 6 percent in men), even when exposed to the same traumas.[11]

Rape is followed by PTSD rates as high as 80 percent, and war is also one of the most important stressors known.[12] The American Psychological Association states that women experience PTSD symptoms longer than men and show more vulnerability to cues that remind them of the trauma.[13] Women, immediately after a traumatic experience, score higher on threat perception and peritraumatic dissociation, a mental process where an individual disconnects from their thoughts, feelings, memories, and sometimes identity.[14] Men tend to cope with traumatic stress through problem-solving, or occasionally by engaging in more reckless or self-destructive activity.[15]

While there is overlap in how men and women experience and respond to trauma, overall women experience more severe symptoms and a longer duration, known as chronicity, compared to men.

POST-TRAUMATIC STRESS DISORDER

Post-traumatic stress disorder (PTSD) is a constellation of symptoms that is remarkably common, affecting millions of Americans and global citizens each year. Despite the prevalence, we still are in the early stages of deeply understanding why some people develop PTSD and why some do not. PTSD is defined as a condition in which a person has trouble recovering after witnessing or experiencing terror, which may entail a range of experiences from war to death of a loved one to rape or abuse (see more examples in the text). It robs one of inner peace and may last months or years. PTSD may never resolve, it may slowly resolve, it may partially resolve, it may fully and completely resolve—and that's where applying art and science to find the most effective solutions, tailored to the individual, becomes essential.

Symptoms feel like the traumatic event continues to occur with intense emotional, psychological, physiological, and physical reactions that run the gamut of nightmares, flashbacks, difficulty sleeping and concentrating, depression, anxiety, and feelings of guilt, shame, irritability, anger, and isolation. While I've listed the medical findings, a person with PTSD has problems far beyond the clinical, including loss of trust, closeness, and communication and diminished problem-solving abilities, leading to difficulty in relationships, unnecessary breakups, separation, divorce, and suicide.

Trauma can damage your body, especially your psychology, immune, neurological, and endocrine networks. Trauma worsens other health conditions, including:

- **PSYCHIATRIC PROBLEMS.** Eighty percent of people with PTSD have another psychiatric diagnosis, such as depression, anxiety, substance use disorder, or dissociation.[16]
- **CHRONIC PAIN.** For example, in one study of eighty-eight women with fibromyalgia, most participants (71.5 percent) met the diagnostic criteria for current post-traumatic stress disorder (PTSD).[17]
- **RHEUMATIC CONDITIONS.** People with two or more adverse childhood experiences have a 100 percent increased risk for rheumatic diseases.[18]
- **AUTOIMMUNE DISEASE.** For instance, bereaved parents of people killed in combat have double the rate of multiple sclerosis compared to controls.[19]
- **CANCER.** Women with PTSD have twice the risk of ovarian cancer.[20]

PTSD is disorienting, and can make a person lose heart and feel utterly disconnected from others; frankly, life may feel unbearable. You don't have to be diagnosed with full-on PTSD to suffer; you might experience partial or sub-threshold PTSD and suffer just as much. We need to be approaching traumatic exposure and PTSD as public health conditions that require a broad and multidisciplinary team to address not just the clinical but the relational, social, and ecological contexts.[21]

Why the Differences?

Why the differences? In particular, why differences in autoimmunity and PTSD? We don't know all the answers but have several theories related to biological and gender (socially constructed) differences, stress response, hormones, and the role of oxytocin and internalization of emotions.

Some of this comes back to social constructions, such as gender differences in quantity, type, and timing of trauma, which contribute to differences in how the body responds. Men encounter more potentially traumatic events, but women are more likely to suffer with long-term consequences.

The type of trauma can be distinct and that difference can matter: men are more likely to encounter physical violence, accidents, terrorist attacks, physical abuse (including as children), and combat; to witness injury or violence and police brutality; and to be subject to state-sponsored or institutional violence and incarceration.[22] Women are exposed to more adversity in childhood, including sexual abuse or rape, intimate partner violence, kidnapping, and stalking at frequencies and levels of disparity so remarkable they are worth a careful look.

Not unrelated, trauma timing is different by gender. According to research, women experience trauma at an earlier age, most commonly sexual abuse in childhood, when they are more vulnerable and have fewer coping strategies to manage trauma and heal. This matters because the risk of PTSD is highest in childhood, in adolescence, and over the age of sixty-five. Dr. Miranda Olff of the University of Amsterdam observes in her recent journal article: "Trauma early in life has more impact, especially when it involves type II trauma (trauma that is prolonged versus type I, also known as single-incident, or impact trauma), interfering with neurobiological development and personality. Traumatic stress affects different areas of the brains of boys and girls at different ages."[23]

The intersection of trauma with race can create even greater burdens for Black women. We know that women who endure more discrimination and marginalization due to racism, health inequity, homophobia, or poverty often experience more cumulative trauma. In racially mixed data sets, Black women experience the highest rates of racial weathering, which is the physiological cost of high-effort coping with chronic stressors from the environment, even when adjusted for socioeconomic status.

It's not just the trauma that you experience—now we know that heritability of trauma in families is higher in women.[24] When intergenerational and collective trauma compounds with racism, we see even more trauma hazards for brown and Black women.[25]

Against this violent tableau, it's no wonder that men have a lower life expectancy and women are shamed out of their bodies at an early age. I think it's the violence turned inward that may be a key factor in the autoimmunity gender gap. Let's look at how the harm travels from outside to inside, from incident to PTSD to autoimmune disease.

Refinery29 performed a survey of one thousand women and found that 65 percent were criticized about their body by age fourteen, and 41 percent were criticized between ages ten and thirteen.[26] Women are told they are not right—too thick, too thin, too hairy, too short, too brown, too big, too aggressive, too much. The trauma of being female in a patriarchal society leads to private suffering and shame. We dissociate from our interior world and stop speaking the truth about our external world. We doubt ourselves and our inner guidance about right and wrong, then we beat ourselves up for not measuring up to impossible standards. *New York Times* bestselling author and poet Cole Arthur Riley recently said on the *We Can Do Hard Things* podcast that we as women get shamed out of our bodies young, and then dissociation makes us stay out of our bodies, almost like a defense mechanism. Then we wonder, *Am I in here?* We don't inhabit our bodies, our own homes. A survivor of ongoing sexual abuse as a child, Cole describes the mercy of being exiled from the body, and how distance creates disdain and, in her case, led to bulimia.[27]

I survived ongoing sexual abuse as a young child. At a time when kids are typically learning how to move in their bodies— discovering their agility, the age that they are learning that they can jump from here to there, learning how to be free—I was learning how to leave my body to survive. That was my strength. To leave my body. I'm certainly no expert, but we know that's a very common, and at times necessary, trauma response. Dissociation gets a bad name, but in the immediacy of the traumatic experience, it's a mercy. Sadly for me and for many other people, it just happens to be that this mercy becomes a habit that extends even when the threat is no longer there anymore. We ex-

WHAT TYPES OF TRAUMA
DISPROPORTIONATELY IMPACT WOMEN?[28]

- One in three women globally, around 736 million, are subjected to physical or sexual violence.[29]
- Twenty-four percent of women experience sexual abuse, according to a study of 22,224 people from sixteen countries.[30] However, only 12 percent of child sexual abuse is reported to the authorities, so prevalence can be difficult to track.[31] According to a global meta-analysis of 217 studies,[32] the highest rates of sexual abuse of girls were found in Australia, whereas the highest rates of sexual abuse of boys were found in Africa. Asia has the lowest rates of sexual abuse of both girls and boys, though my Asian colleagues counsel me not to trust the low numbers.
- One in five women and one in seventy-one men will be raped during their lives. According to the Rape, Abuse & Incest National Network in the United States, rape is the most underreported crime: 63 percent of sexual assaults are not reported to police. Only 12 percent of child sexual abuse is reported to the authorities.[33]
- Eight to 24 percent of women will be stalked by someone over their lifetime, either known or unknown to them.[34] The average is one in six women; for men it is one in nineteen.
- Intimate partner violence is 2.3-fold higher in women compared to men[35] and is associated with high PTSD risk.[36]
- Women who endure more discrimination and marginalization due to racism, health inequity, homophobia, and poverty often experience more cumulative trauma. In racially mixed data sets, Black women experience the highest rates of racial weathering (defined originally by Arline Geronimus, ScD, a public health researcher at the University of Michigan, as the cumulative racism experienced by Black women that causes them to experience inferior outcomes compared to other races and even Black men), a finding that remains even when adjusted for socioeconomic status.

All of these variables add up to social, economic, psychological, and interpersonal victimization that becomes cumulative and erosive.

tend it. And I think that happened for both my grandma and me. We begin dissociating even when we don't want to and we don't necessarily need to for survival. I was already at a distance from my body, and that was my gift. To escape.

Then as I go into adolescence and my dance training picks up, I'm in front of a mirror for hours every day, and I can't escape the sight of my own face. I can't escape the relationship with my body. So what do I do? I turn against it. What once was just distance or departure, became disdain, self-hatred. I mean, maybe it begins with neglect, but it ends with self-hatred. For me, I think that is the story of my bulimia. A hatred of my body. But more than that, a hatred of the inescapability of myself, which I think is so sinister. It's so imprecise but that new ritual of purging, that hatred of the body, felt so necessary to my survival in the same way that leaving my body felt necessary to my survival. The desire to leave became a desire to annihilate.

Cole describes a common response to trauma, dissociation, as a mercy, not a bad thing. I agree. She then turned against her body in disdain, in annihilation, in how she fed herself. Psychiatrist Stephen Porges, MD, frames the development of eating disorders like bulimia within his polyvagal theory; that is, an eating disorder can occur when eating behavior replaces social behavior as a regulator of the nervous system. That feels right and relevant to my own disordered eating and also potentially relevant to the central role in autoimmunity of turning against oneself.

Why Do Women Experience More PTSD?

We pick up again with Dr. Olff, who further explains how this trauma-based turn on the body changes physiology, providing additional catalysts for PTSD and the autoimmune response. Here, we move more toward sex differences, even as we don't lose contact with gender dynamics entirely. Dr. Olff especially homes in on the roles of the hypothalamic-pituitary-adrenal (HPA) axis and everyone's favorite hormone (oxytocin). Interestingly, in the problem may lie the cure. Let's see.

- **HYPOTHALAMIC-PITUITARY-ADRENAL (HPA) AXIS.** The way that your body responds to stress in terms of producing cortisol via the HPA axis is more sensitive in women. As a

result, women with traumatic stress that jacks up the HPA
axis may find that they have more circadian disruption,
including sleep issues, compared to men.[37] In turn, circadian
disruption and sleep disturbance increase the risk of PTSD.
On the other hand, men have a more sensitive arousal system,
which generally can increase alertness, elevate heart rate, and
rapidly respire, responses that are not linked to the HPA axis
and circadian disruption.[38] Overall, the difference in the HPA
axis leads to a difference in fear systems as part of the overall
sex-specific PTSD vulnerability. Fear, an adaptive response
buried deep in the body and genes, becomes pathological in
PTSD.[39]

- **EFFECTS OF OXYTOCIN.** Females experience and respond
  to toxic stress differently and have evolved distinct ways to
  support their unique physiology. Oxytocin, the hormone
  of attachment and love, present in both men and women,
  buffers the effects of traumatic stress.[40] Oxytocin is
  produced in the hypothalamus, a part of the brain involved
  in hormonal control. Normally, females have higher levels
  of oxytocin than males because females are often more
  communicative and socially connected, plus our higher
  estrogen levels enable the production of more oxytocin.
  Trauma may decrease oxytocin and oxytocin receptors in
  childhood and adulthood.[41] Therein lies both a blessing and a
  curse: oxytocin and connection with others can help females
  survive trauma with less mental and physical damage, but
  that reliance on the support of others during traumatic stress
  can also work against women if the social network is not
  able to provide adequate support. Women do best when they
  can tend and befriend under traumatic stress—tending or
  caretaking people in our orbit, and befriending or reaching
  out to others to process what's happened. In other words,
  women seek social support more than men and it raises
  oxytocin, but lack of social support is a consistent predictor of
  a negative outcome from trauma.[42] When women feel rejected
  or abandoned, oxytocin may be lower and they may be more
  vulnerable to PTSD.

These changes in the HPA axis and oxytocin play a role in the reactive cascades of the PINE system and inflammation that underlie autoimmune disease, as previously discussed.

What to Do?

Given the escalating rates of trauma and autoimmunity, it's pressing to ask, are there ways that men and women heal from trauma differently? Even as the evidence of a strong case for heightened concern for women with regard to autoimmunity does not diminish male trauma, we need to take care to understand the range of experiences and how men and women may need different trauma-informed treatment.[43] For example, some evidence indicates that women benefit more than men from psychotherapy to reduce PTSD symptoms.[44] Circadian disruption and sleep disturbance increase the risk of PTSD, and suggest that humans, but perhaps even more, women, may need more study of biological rhythms for trauma recovery, such as early morning light.[45] Can we work around the toxic stress issue by giving you oxytocin, and would it help men as much as women? Maybe, as we will explore in a later chapter.

Wrap-Up

Our world is a hot mess. If you find it traumatizing, you are not alone. You may be having a sane reaction to insane events. Violence and trauma are so pervasive that we are all affected, either directly or indirectly, even as violence and trauma hit women differently, making them increasingly a women's health issue. This creates an endless loop of harm, and unless the trauma is healed, traumatic stress can cause many health problems besides autoimmunity, including depression, anxiety, and post-traumatic stress disorder. Not all who survive trauma will have mental or physical dysregulation, but women are more likely to than men.

Emotional trauma is more common in women, and women are more likely to suffer from long-term consequences. Certainly, men have a unique experience in response to trauma too—more problem-solving and reckless behavior, but also less shame and negative feelings about themselves.

While I cannot take away all of your fear in this book, my goal is for you to learn about normal fear versus pathological fear, so that we can locate the origins of the pathological fear and transmute it into a feeling that serves your body better.

In the upcoming chapters, we will unearth the healing strategies that seem to be the most effective. As we do, keep in mind the words of my friend and colleague Will Van Derveer, MD, co-founder of Integrative Psychiatry Institute: "As a psychiatrist, I learned early in my career that a psychological approach to mental health is incomplete. Similarly, a purely physical approach is incomplete. Further, a spiritual approach is incomplete. We need to address all areas of well-being." Dr. Van Derveer and I agree that by combining the best of personalized medicine with psychedelic medicine, we have the best opportunity for re-creating wholeness and health.

CHAPTER 5

Why Pharmaceuticals and Talk Therapy May Not Be Enough

Most of us brought up in the tradition of western medical science tend to regard illness as a kind of mechanical breakdown that afflicts our bodies and requires a technical repair. The physician becomes the mechanic under the hood and a cure is something done to and for us.

—BILL MOYERS, "HEALING FROM WITHIN," *HEALING AND THE MIND* TV SERIES, FEBRUARY 23, 1993

I n 2011, when I was writing my first book, *The Hormone Cure*, I was shocked to learn how many hormonal problems were being treated with a completely wrong approach: pharmaceuticals for mental health. I was surprised to find that one in four women received this treatment (or should we call it "mistreatment"?). Then I was disturbed. Then outraged. It's not normal to have a population in which one in four women are taking pills for their mental health, and, more importantly, it's not helping. It's not just our mental health that suffers because of this epidemic of excess prescription. So do the autoimmunity and unresolved trauma—the root cause of the issues—which are never addressed.

Women aren't the only ones who are overmedicated: 25 percent of adolescents and one in six American adults are taking psychiatric medications. Of course, sometimes medication is needed, especially if it's used alongside the slow process of trauma resolution that utilizes a range of modalities. But on the whole, it seems too many people are taking too many pills that aren't truly helping them. And how did we get here?

As I trained to become a physician, I was taught to diagnose a patient with a problem and then offer a pill. I got very good at it, as comfortable as that seasoned car mechanic under the hood. I wasn't alone. Many doctors hope that prescribing a pharmaceutical will help a patient be or feel normal. And it's easier for a clinician to write a prescription than to roll up the sleeves and get to the hard work of plumbing the depths of the psyche and individual healing. It's not just the clinicians either. We're all busy, and many patients accept, and sometimes prefer, the option of a pill to the more challenging and confronting work of addressing trauma-driven behaviors, like eating processed foods, bingeing on drama, or raging at their spouse.

Then I realized the flaws with this approach.

First, we all have an innate ability to heal. The codependent relationship with pills that we've been sold can bypass our inner healing intelligence, the principle that we all can access to perpetually restore, regain equilibrium, and move toward wholeness and health.[1]

Second, pharmaceutical methods are based on populations, not individuals. The "pill for the ill" is the same regardless of the patient's specific circumstances, and the result is medicine for the average, not the individual.

Third, pills block biochemistry to reduce symptoms, which leads to side effects and other problems.

Fourth, there's so much more uncertainty about medicating illness than mainstream medicine or pharmaceutical companies want to admit. This is especially true regarding trauma and autoimmunity as well as conditions like chronic Lyme disease, fibromyalgia, chronic fatigue syndrome, and biotoxin illness (also known as chronic inflammatory response syndrome, which can flare up when someone is exposed to mold).[2]

Fifth, and this is an emerging concept that I love to discuss with my colleagues in psychedelic medicine: ordinary states of consciousness may not allow you to heal at the deepest level, where the hurt is.

Finally, no pill cures trauma or its consequences, such as an imbalanced immune system that may lead to autoimmunity.

We need a novel approach. True and lasting healing requires a different way of working with your psychological and biological material, in a way that incorporates the wisdom of the body, rather than skipping over it.

In this chapter, we'll explore why conventional medicine for trauma and autoimmunity doesn't work most of the time and consider the latest evidence-based recommendations and novel treatments. We'll explore the history of pills for trauma and autoimmunity and what the science shows, and introduce a better approach committed to your personal growth and expansion. I'll explain the value of contacting your pain and discomfort so that you can access them as a tool for growth, rather than trying to steamroll over them with a pill. Most importantly, by the end of the chapter, I'd love for you to understand the imperative to consider the trauma you may have stored in the body. Men do this more commonly than women. Untreated trauma has deadly consequences.

A History of Pill Pushing

Have you been prescribed any of the following medications?

- Sertraline (Zoloft)
- Paroxetine (Paxil)
- Fluoxetine (Prozac)
- Venlafaxine (Effexor)
- Nefazodone (Serzone)
- Imipramine (Tofranil)
- Phenelzine (Nardil)
- Olanzapine (Zyprexa)
- Quetiapine (Seroquel)
- Buspirone (Buspar)
- Risperidone (Risperdal)
- Lorazepam (Ativan)
- Clonazepam (Klonopin)

- Alprazolam (Xanax)
- Diazepam (Valium)

These pharmaceuticals are prescribed for a wide range of conditions, such as anxiety, depression, obsessive-compulsive disorder, premenstrual syndrome, premenstrual dysphoric disorder, hot flashes, mania, and post-traumatic stress disorder (PTSD). But today's meds actually come from a long history of pill pushing: Looking back to the way that we have treated depression, the first pharmaceutical approved by the Federal Drug Administration in 1933 is in a drug class with many constituents considered illegal today—amphetamines (in this case, intranasal), so-called uppers. Then came lithium, which, for perspective, is a drug for mood stabilization. Other medications followed—chlorpromazine, imipramine, reserpine, and clozapine in the 1950s. Fast-forward to the 1980s, and that's when buproprion and fluoxetine, the first selective serotonin reuptake inhibitors, were approved.

Not coincidentally, there's a rising bottom line that contours this rise in prescriptions. To be blunt, there is big money in pharmaceuticals: Pfizer, the maker of sertraline (Zoloft), has a market capitalization of $267 billion; for Eli Lilly, manufacturer of olanzapine (Zyprexa), that figure is $334 billion. There hadn't been many novel therapies until intranasal ketamine (esketamine) was approved in 2019, following a number of studies on other psychedelic therapies like MDMA and psilocybin for PTSD and depression. (We will talk more about these treatments later in the book.)

The list above features the latest treatments for PTSD, either short or long term, which affects ten million people in the United States alone. The old way of dealing with trauma was to give a trauma survivor a downer like an antianxiety pill (an example is alprazolam, or Xanax). Then we prescribed antidepressants: now four of them are FDA approved for PTSD. In fairness, there has been some improvement. According to the Department of Veterans Affairs website and the 2017 Veterans Affairs/Department of Defense Clinical Practice Guideline for PTSD, trauma-focused psychotherapy is considered the first-line treatment for PTSD rather than pharmacotherapy, but even so, for patients who prefer a pill or don't have access to trauma-focused psychotherapy (many), pills are a treatment option.[3] I submit, though, that this guideline is out-of-date, having been developed prior to the recent groundbreaking publications on and increasing promise of MDMA-assisted therapy, which has had significantly more success in durably treating PTSD.[4]

So many of us in the United States are taking a medication from the previous list for our mental health. As mentioned, one in four women take a psychiatric medication, compared to only 12 percent of women who have received therapy in the past twelve months, according to a survey from 2020.[5] Men are less likely to default to this option: 15 percent are on a medication for mental health versus 8 percent who have received counseling or therapy. Still, men also suffer, and their trauma has major impacts. The gender gap suggests women are potentially more vulnerable, more pathologized, more likely to be overprescribed psychotropic medication for hormonal changes like perimenopause, and/or are more likely to seek help.[6] The high numbers have been consistent for the past decade,[7] and rates of use continue to increase in women but not men.[8]

But do they work?

There are many ways to answer this question, but let's examine them through the lens of trauma, since the focus of this book is on the nexus of trauma and autoimmunity. In medicine, we consider all of these pills to be low in effectiveness for treating PTSD.[9] A recent systematic review and meta-analysis of 115 trials showed the current top five medications—fluoxetine, paroxetine, sertraline, venlafaxine, and, less so, quetiapine—have sound evidence that they lower PTSD symptoms, but the magnitude of effect is modest.[10] Sometimes a second drug is added to treat PTSD, but the authors found added benefit is minimal.[11]

One way to assess the effectiveness of a pharmaceutical is the number needed to treat (NNT). According to a systematic review of selective serotonin reuptake inhibitors, or SSRIs (like sertraline, paroxetine, and fluoxetine from the list above), for patients with depression, the NNT is seven.[12] That means that a clinician would need to prescribe an SSRI to seven depressed patients and only one of the seven (14 percent) would improve more than if all seven were given a placebo. Sobering news for many—that these pills are less effective than they may have previously thought—and most of the trials were sponsored by pharmaceutical companies, throwing into doubt any findings of effectiveness. Other studies have confirmed the strong placebo effect (meaning people get better through the power of their minds rather than the action of the pill) and low treatment efficacy of pharmaceuticals for depression and other maladies.[13]

When there's such a long list of PTSD pharmaceuticals available, and they don't clearly work well or at all to solve the problem you're facing, we have to consider that we haven't yet articulated the problem correctly and may be treating the wrong thing and in the wrong way. Most pills work by blocking the normal biochemistry in the body. When emotions and psychic wounds are driving the biochemistry, it's unlikely that blocking the usual chemical reactions is going to solve the problem that's causing symptoms. It may help with symptom management, but it usually doesn't address the root cause, and the patient continues to suffer.

What about pharmaceuticals to dampen the immune system in autoimmune conditions? Results are similar, but there's the added complexity of walking a tightrope with the immune system between risk and harm. Let's examine rheumatoid arthritis (RA) as an example. The main treatment for RA is methotrexate, which blocks an enzyme in the nutritional pathway of folic acid, and therefore suppresses the immune system by decreasing DNA synthesis, repair, and cell replication. NNT is seven for a 50 percent response rate at one year (i.e., seven patients would need to be treated for just one of them to have a 50 percent improvement).[14] Another treatment given with methotrexate is a common biologic agent called rituximab, a drug that depletes B cells in the immune system with a monoclonal antibody; it has an NNT of six.[15] Other reviews have confirmed comparable results,[16] and with other biologic agents.[17] Overall, biologic agents have an NNT of twelve in RA for reducing progression of joint destruction on X-ray.[18] Also of note: side effects from immune suppressants are common, like less resistance to infection and potentially cancer, poor wound healing, glucose problems, weight gain, menstrual irregularity, cholesterol issues, and cortisol dysregulation.[19]

Of course, there's a crossover effect too: sometimes the symptoms of autoimmune disease, like fatigue, poor sleep, and mood dysfunction, are treated with psychiatric medications. The same inflammation pathways that harm your thyroid or joints or gut may also cause your mental health to decline. We'll explore the connection between mental and physical health, including the spectrum of symptoms, more in chapter 7.

There is a time and a place for pharmaceutical treatment to manage symptoms. You may have been prescribed antidepressants, antianxiety medications, stimulants, antipsychotics, mood stabilizers, sleeping pills, and immunosuppressants for trauma or even autoimmune disease—and found them helpful, even lifesaving or life enhancing in some situations. While it can require a greater effort to stabilize mental illness and autoimmune disease without pharmaceutical treatment, that's not the best choice for everyone. I advocate the middle path. I am not against pharmaceuticals. I've written many thousands of prescriptions, but decades of experience, which statistics confirm, have shown me that the way I was taught to prescribe is excessive. I do far less prescribing now—I write about 75 percent fewer prescriptions—compared to twenty years ago. Much of the excessive prescribing has a profit motive driven by the pharmaceutical industry, and let's face it, they are not necessarily interested in you healing and getting off their latest patented blockbuster drug.

Yet untreated mental illness and autoimmune disease have serious consequences, including greater stress, worsening function, disability, poor quality of life, loss of relationships, unemployment, and suicide. The key is to suss out with your clinician the best option given your current circumstances. You will need to consider your history, your diagnosis, the symptoms you're experiencing, and your risk of relapse of symptoms. If you've tried lifestyle medicine for some time and you continue to worsen or hit a plateau, a pharmaceutical may help and could be approached as an experiment. If your symptoms are severe or worsening, or if you cannot function in your daily activities, you may need temporary pharmaceutical support. The main takeaway: sometimes drugs can help, but not always. My advice is to do the full menu of work that helps you heal, and pharmaceuticals may be part of that plan when necessary.

How Well Does Talk Therapy Work?

In the same way that many patients who struggle with autoimmune symptoms such as anxiety, depression, and sleep disruption end up getting prescribed psychiatric medications, many also try talk therapy (also known simply as therapy or counseling). It helps some but not all. Many barriers to therapy exist, such as high cost, long waits to initiate care, long waits to see progress, and an ongoing commitment. Further, according to my colleague psychiatrist Will Van Derveer, MD, patients with high inflammation levels are more likely to be resistant to talk therapy—and most people with autoimmune disease have high levels of inflammation. Given what we know about inflammation, we believe that people without inflammation are probably the ones most likely to benefit from talk therapy. Dr. Van Derveer prefers integrative anti-inflammatory treatments in these patients, such as ketamine or low-dose naltrexone. (We will explore these integrative treatments and novel modulators of the immune response in more detail in chapters 10 and 12.)

In fact, talk therapy may not actually be designed for trauma. Most talk therapy is a "top-down" cognitive-based approach that encourages you to become more aware of your most troublesome thoughts while learning how to change them through thinking and speaking about them. While this may help some people with anxiety or depression, it doesn't work well for trauma. Recognition of this problem has led to a different approach for PTSD that is more "bottom-up." This trauma-informed care honors the wisdom of the body's sensations to access trauma held in tissues as opposed to the more conventional cognitive approach. We are in the early stages of this shift to trauma-informed care, trauma-informed education, and trauma-informed approaches not just to mental health but to physical health as well. As my friend Lissa Rankin, MD, recently wrote, "It is my sincere prayer that our institutions wake up and prioritize including an integrated, trauma-informed approach to all of our systems in medicine, psychology, education, law enforcement, finance, government, environmentalism, and social justice activism."[20] Yes, please.

Bessel van der Kolk, MD, a psychiatrist specializing in trauma, explains why talk therapy isn't enough for PTSD: understanding and feeling are located in different parts of the brain.[21] While a person may understand their trauma, their feelings need to emerge and be processed to get results. Consequently, talking about a traumatic experience and recounting the events doesn't seem to help much in people with PTSD. He says that therapists are usually insufficiently trauma-trained, guiding clients down paths that fail to yield healing. For those of us with trauma, the event itself is in the past and does not need to be described in detail to a therapist. As Dr. van der Kolk puts it, "Telling the story is not helpful." According to him, talking and purely cognitive approaches do not sufficiently help people heal, but expanded states of consciousness, such as with psychedelic-assisted therapy, just might.

I agree. I've seen about a dozen or more therapists in the past thirty-five years, have divulged in exquisite detail my experiences of trauma, and have found it mostly unhelpful. Understanding did not change my feelings, though it may help some people. Retelling the story just seemed to reinforce my cognitive understanding of what happened, but it didn't get to the depth of my feelings in a separate part of my brain. In contrast, psychedelic-assisted therapy helped me metabolize my trauma and change my behaviors—and seems to have resolved my high antinuclear antibodies—as we will discuss further in Part 2.

What gives? Traditional talk therapy mostly ignores the body, where the trauma is lodged, and many people commonly drop out of treatment before they are fully recovered. Increasingly, mental health and other clinicians believe that somatic therapy may be the key to healing trauma and stress disorders. "Somatic therapy" refers to a type of treatment that is "of, relating to, or affecting the body." Traumatized people can feel trapped by their past experience, unable to break free of the suffering because their body-based biological systems get disrupted. Somatic therapy can help as it integrates one's awareness of internal bodily experience, including sensations, energy, movements, gestures, and body postures. Somatics provide a way to use breath, touch, and body awareness as a vehicle to deepen and transform psychological experience in a nonverbal language.

After spending a small fortune on top-down cognitive approaches in talk therapy, I didn't feel any better. Trauma was still driving much of my experience—chronic burnout from overwork and conflict with my family. Then I began seeing a Hakomi therapist, which is a type of somatic therapy. I was hooked because it unlocked psychological states that got trapped in my body and unwound old patterns from childhood that I was still experiencing, bringing them to my mindful attention to be processed with my somatic therapist. You will learn more about Hakomi in chapter 11.

If traditional mental health approaches are at best modestly effective, why is mainstream medicine in such a rush to prescribe drugs and standard psychotherapy for trauma and its sequelae, when they don't seem to be enough?

Emotions are mysterious. In response to a particular internal and external environment, your emotional reaction may spiral to extremes, potentially leading to declining mental and physical health. Sometimes the mystery can get lost in a rush to label and pathologize emotional difficulties, and we may lack an invitation to navigate and feel the emotionality through to completion. Think of it as *medicalization*, a process in which authentic human experience is deemed pathological in origin and treated as a medical condition.

Medical psychiatry is mostly based on the idea that psychological and emotional problems are linked to changes in biology, like levels of neurotransmitters or certain patterns of brain activity. The converse is likewise assumed: that symptom resolution changes biology. However, mental health difficulties may not always be biological in origin. It may be true of certain mental illness, like schizophrenia, compared to others. But always assuming mental illness is biological in origin may be overly reductionistic.

Reading a luminous book by Meghan O'Rourke, *The Invisible Kingdom: Reimagining Chronic Illness*, I was struck by something she noticed that always bothered me about mainstream medicine: stress is considered something measurable and observable, whereas trauma is considered something psychological requiring a referral to a psychiatrist or therapist. Yet, as I keep emphasizing in this book, *both stress and trauma initiate similar pathways in the body that can harm homeostasis*. We need clinicians and methodologies that understand this concept and can work through it with you.

We Need an Integrative Approach

Hakomi is not the only way to work with what you hold in the body. Other methods can also help you notice the ongoing interactions between your body and mind, and they color your daily experience of triggers. Some are more evidence-based than others. Regardless, there have not been reports of dangerous side effects with these treatments and my advice is to find a practitioner with many years of experience who feels like a good fit and is certified in the technique. Here are the additional methods.

- **SOMATIC EXPERIENCING (SE)** is a body-oriented model of therapy to help heal trauma and other stress disorders. It was developed by psychologist Peter Levine after witnessing that prey animals recover from trauma by physically releasing the energy that accumulates in their body during stress, such as with shaking or trembling to discharge their burden and return to a calm state. From the Somatic Experiencing website (see Resources), SE helps to resolve "stress, shock, and trauma that accumulate in our bodies. When we are stuck in patterns of fight, flight, or freeze, SE helps us release, recover, and become more resilient."

- **SENSORIMOTOR PSYCHOTHERAPY**, developed by psychotherapist Pat Ogden to specifically heal the impact of attachment trauma, is a hybrid of somatic therapy, attachment theory, neuroscience, cognitive approaches, and techniques from Hakomi. It integrates cognitive and somatic techniques.

- **EYE MOVEMENT DESENSITIZATION AND REPROCESSING (EMDR)** was developed by Francine Shapiro in 1987 when she observed that walking in the forest and scanning laterally with her eyes to the right and left of the forest floor seemed to make her own difficult memories less troubling. In this method, you focus on a traumatic memory while paying attention to a back-and-forth movement or sound until shifts occur in the way that you experience the memory. While it can assist in healing PTSD, there is disagreement about how it works.[22] You will find that EMDR is recommended by organizations such as the American Psychological Association (APA) and the World Health Organization (WHO).

- **NEURO EMOTIONAL TECHNIQUE (NET)** is a research-supported method to assist in the release and resolution of past traumas and unresolved stress. It's not counseling or psychotherapy but a mind-body stress reduction technique that we use regularly at the Marcus Institute of Integrative Health in Pennsylvania, where I work. It addresses the physiology or physical aspects of emotionally charged stress responses. The goal of NET is to find and correct the physical aberration, not the emotions.

- **POLYVAGAL THEORY**, developed by Stephen Porges, MD, acknowledges that shifts in the autonomic nervous system produce three elementary states—rest-and-digest (social and safe), fight-or-flight (mobilization), and shutdown (immobilization)—that can function as a ladder. Polyvagal theory offers coregulation (an interactive process of regulatory support, explored more in the next chapter) as a method that engages the social nervous system of the therapist and client.

- **MINDFULNESS-BASED STRESS REDUCTION (MBSR)** was originally designed as a form of natural medicine for stress management, but it can be used to treat many conditions, including but not limited to PTSD, depression, anxiety, immune disorders, diabetes, disordered eating, and chronic pain.[23] MBSR can help if you tend toward having difficulty quieting your mind during meditation: when a thought floats into your consciousness, you observe it, label it, and gently let it go, without getting caught up or feeling guilty about it. For instance, while meditating, if you start thinking about your dinner, you tell yourself something like "planning for the future," and let it go. As you become more proficient at this, you become less attached to your thoughts, and thus less reactive. In short, MBSR promotes awareness of the present moment with a compassionate, nonjudgmental stance, which over time leads to a shift in perception and response. MBSR increases activity in the part of the brain that governs learning and memory while decreasing activity in the area responsible for worry and fear. Not surprisingly, MBSR lowers cortisol, improves sleep, decreases worry, and reduces depression, anxiety, and distress in people with various stress-related health problems.[24] There is a trauma-informed version of MBSR.[25]

- **GESTALT** is not specifically a trauma therapy, but a holistic approach focused on the present moment rather than past experiences. Founded in the 1950s, Gestalt embraces the "paradoxical theory of change," which posits that people heal when they become deeply aware of who they are, not trying to become someone else. It is centered on increasing your awareness, freedom, and self-direction.

- **BRAINSPOTTING** was developed in 2003 by David Grand, PhD. The idea is that there are points in the client's visual field, called brain spots, that may help to access unprocessed trauma in the subcortical brain. The brainspotting therapist uses relevant eye positions to locate, focus, process, and release emotionality, trauma, and other body-based conditions, such as those related to performance and resilience. It is a brain-based tool that can support the therapeutic relationship. In the words of Dr. Grand: "Where you look affects how you feel." According to proponents, it is the brain activity in the subcortical brain that organizes itself around that eye position.

- **OTHER SOMATIC EXERCISES** include emotional freedom technique (tapping), rolfing, body-mind centering, Alexander Technique, Feldenkrais Method, Laban Movement Analysis, somatic bodywork, and sexological bodywork.

- **TWELVE-STEP PROGRAMS** are not therapy and are not considered a treatment, but they are a free or low-cost option for some people to support recovery from substance use disorders (such as alcohol and drugs) and behavioral addictions and compulsions (not just gambling, but food and sex too). It was originally developed in the 1930s as Alcoholics Anonymous (AA) to help overcome alcoholism, and since then dozens of similar organizations have applied the AA approach to other matters. Potential side effects can occur with any of these treatments, therapies, or organizations. Working with trauma can make one feel uncomfortable and awkward, especially at the beginning. One may feel challenged to share private feelings and thoughts, but a lack of disclosure and vulnerability can hinder treatment. Note that methods like EMDR are designed to help a person reprocess difficult memories. This may result in intense emotions, new and additional memories, even significant distress. What's happening under the hood is that brain networks may be destabilized in order to create new pathways that are healthier.

We will explore in more detail a few of these modalities that I've found to be particularly helpful in chapter 11, "Mind-Body Therapy Protocol."

But there is more, and when combined with something from the above list, more may be better—much better.

Out of all of the treatments described in this chapter, there is one integrative approach that seems to outperform the rest: *MDMA-assisted therapy*. In this approach, MDMA, a stimulant also known by its street names of Molly or Ecstasy, is prescribed in specific psychotherapy sessions to improve treatment effectiveness. Multiple randomized trials show that MDMA can improve psychotherapy by lowering defensiveness, anxiety, and fear; modulating the reconsolidation of memories of fear; improving mood and increasing relaxation. It works by triggering serotonin release and possibly oxytocin. Six randomized trials have been published showing safety and effectiveness at phase two trials.[26] The phase three data, published in the prestigious journal *Nature Medicine*, indicate that in patients with PTSD, MDMA-assisted therapy induced significant improvement in symptoms on a PTSD scale known as the Clinician-Administered PTSD Scale (CAPS-5, the primary endpoint of the study). The authors write: "These data indicate that, compared with manualized therapy with inactive placebo, MDMA-assisted therapy is highly efficacious in individuals with severe PTSD, and treatment is safe and well-tolerated, even in those with comorbidities. We conclude that MDMA-assisted therapy represents a potential breakthrough treatment that merits expedited clinical evaluation."[27]

While the pharmaceuticals we reviewed earlier in this chapter, such as selective serotonin reuptake inhibitors, have a low effect size in reducing PTSD compared to placebo (quantified as a standardized mean difference of -0.28, meaning there may be a 25 percent improvement),[28] MDMA-assisted therapy has an effect size that is 3.89 times greater (standardized mean difference -1.09), according to a systematic review and meta-analysis of twenty-one randomized, controlled trials.[29] That means MDMA-assisted therapy has the potential to be nearly fourfold better in treating PTSD, and recent phase three trials have confirmed that it's not only effective, but that the benefits are durable for years after treatment. So you don't go to weekly talk therapy—instead you have three preparatory sessions and an MDMA-assisted journey with two therapists, followed by three integration sessions. And if you had PTSD at the beginning, two out of three subjects will no longer meet criteria for PTSD by the end of the last integration session.

In another recent systematic review and meta-analysis from researchers in the United Kingdom, six different nonpharmacological approaches emerged with growing evidence: acupuncture, neurofeedback, saikokei-shikankyoto (an herbal preparation), somatic experiencing, transcranial magnetic stimulation, and yoga.[30] While these do not yet have sufficient evidence to be first-line treatments for PTSD, the existing evidence of efficacy suggests they could be reasonable alternatives for people who do not want or fail to respond fully to conventional approaches—and they may well be excellent complements to MDMA therapy.

Wrap-Up

We've explored the reasons why traditional treatments, cognitive-based, top-down talk therapy and pharmaceuticals, are unlikely to resolve trauma or its consequences, like autoimmunity. Currently, trauma, biological and emotional dysregulation, and an unbalanced immune system are problems without a solution, according to mainstream medicine. *Got trauma? See a psychiatrist.* But that approach may not work as often as you may presume. At best, the effect is modest, with about 30 percent of people experiencing benefit from talk therapy or a pharmaceutical, though trauma-informed therapy may show better outcomes.

Our task is to rebuild homeostasis, starting in the body with a somatic approach and body awareness—and MDMA. Then we can layer in additional novel therapies as needed, like a nourishing and regulating way of eating, sleeping, and creating better balance in the immune, nervous, and endocrine systems.

Consider it a pilgrimage, a journey into an unknown space where our search for deeper meanings about self, others, and human nature combine with the goal of healing trauma by re-creating wholeness.

PART 2

··

REINTEGRATING
THE WHOLE
The Gottfried Protocol

CHAPTER 6

Body Awareness

Integration arises from intimacy with our emotions and our bodies, as well as with our thoughts.

—SHARON SALZBERG, *REAL LOVE: THE ART OF MINDFUL CONNECTION*

I hear from so many of my clients that they have been eating well, carefully managing their stress levels, exercising, and taking the right supplements and herbs—but still feel sick. Deep fatigue, chronic pain, and other mysterious and often invisible symptoms. Time after time, the missing link in their healing journey is *embodiment*, defined as the "lived experience of engagement of the body with the world."[1] This concept might be new to you, as it often is to my patients—but it has always been important not only to your process of healing, but to your own personal journey as well.

It wasn't until my fifties that I learned how to become fully embodied, which for me meant having the ability to notice subtle shifts in my body. I had to unlearn patterns of childhood and early adulthood that taught me to ignore bodily sensations. I had to recognize that dismissing the body was part of the indoctrination I received during my medical training—medical students stop eating at normal mealtimes, don't have the luxury to go to the bathroom when needed, are deprived of sleep, dress in a weird uniform that makes them part of the group (not an individual), and get cut off from the friends and family who help one feel human. I had to come to terms with the added challenges brought by balancing career and family. When you put in a long day at work and come home famished to a busy household—your babysitter trying to escape your home as quickly as possible, your kids fighting, your partner wondering what's for dinner—you must deal with them all regardless of what your body says.

Embodiment is a crucial part of our innate intelligence that can be tapped for healing (i.e., the inner power that governs organization and homeostasis, or balance, throughout all bodily systems). Research suggests that positive embodiment maps to several important dimensions of health, though for our purposes you can frame it as body comfort, agency and function, experience and expression of bodily desires, attuned self-care, and the feeling of "being there."[2] Even short periods of increased body awareness can be healing. On the other hand, when you ignore, neglect, or abuse the maintenance of the body, you are at risk for experiencing more fatigue, burnout, pain, and maybe a shorter healthspan—meaning fewer years of your life that you feel magnificent and brimming with energy.

When you discount the signals of the body for so long, your body may just give up or give out. It can capitulate to the constant cognitive override. The grind of stress and nonstop emergency chemicals can hijack the state of peace that might allow you to tune in to somatic truth.

But by the same token, your body can also be the greatest tool of healing in your arsenal—if you are able to listen to its whispers.

Embodiment Questionnaire

Before we start to investigate and deepen your body awareness, it's important to know about your current experience in your body. Are you connected deeply to your inner landscape, or do you struggle like I used to?

While there are many ways to measure embodiment in research,[3] here are the core prompts that I use to assess level of embodiment in my clients and myself. I hope you will find them helpful as you explore your body awareness. Please read each prompt carefully and then circle one of the numbers to the right to indicate how often you've experienced that quality in the past month. Rate each quality on a scale of one (not at all) to five (consistently).

I feel safe in my body.	1	2	3	4	5
I trust the sensations in my body related to thirst, hunger, and rest.	1	2	3	4	5
I can feel when my body is satisfied with food and heed the cues of hunger and fullness.	1	2	3	4	5
When I feel the need to urinate or defecate, I go to the bathroom within five minutes.	1	2	3	4	5
When I feel discomfort or pain in my body, I stop activity that worsens it.	1	2	3	4	5
I have an intimate connection with my breath, and return to mindful breathing throughout the day.	1	2	3	4	5
I love my body size and shape.	1	2	3	4	5
I feel sexual desire regularly and am satisfied with how I meet my sexual needs.	1	2	3	4	5
I tune into and follow my gut instincts.	1	2	3	4	5
I feel, name, and live with a full spectrum of emotions and sensations as important guides.	1	2	3	4	5
It's easy for me to close my eyes and tune into my inner world and sensations.	1	2	3	4	5
I can feel when my resting heart rate is in my baseline range, and notice when it increases due to my environment (threat, exercise, etc.).	1	2	3	4	5

I know how to stay within my window of tolerance and feel like I can deal with whatever is happening in my life. I may encounter stress, but it doesn't bother me too much.	1	2	3	4	5
I rarely numb out with work, stress, social media, or other addictive tendencies.	1	2	3	4	5
I can use positive and negative feelings in my body to influence decisions and don't need to always use cognition to weigh the pros and cons (i.e., make an intellectual choice).	1	2	3	4	5
I return again and again to my body-based experience of life, as it's from that felt sense that I feel most at peace.	1	2	3	4	5

Scoring. Tally your total from each prompt. A **score of less than forty-five** suggests that embodiment is a challenge for you, and that we have significant work together to support your experience.

A **score of forty-five to sixty-four** indicates that the link between your bodily states, emotions, behaviors, and cognition is moderate but could use reinforcement. A **score of more than sixty-five** indicates you have developed a high degree of embodiment, so keep reading to provide additional attention and awareness to your bodily sensations.

The Shift Toward Inner Noticing

If your score on the questionnaire indicates that embodiment is at least somewhat challenging for you, it's possible that awareness of your body has been shocked out of you, like it was for me. Perhaps you learned to ignore the body and to think instead. You learned to postpone what your body needs or wants. You became adept at keeping your distance from the inner landscape.

The consequences of losing awareness can be wide-ranging. Perhaps your mind doesn't trust the messages that come from the body, or your body doesn't trust your mind to respond to them appropriately. Perhaps you override the body's urgings and tend to overeat, overindulge, stay in bed, or zone out on the couch watching television.

For me, the experience of shutting down my body awareness has left a legacy. I grind my teeth at night and must remind myself daily to release tension in my jaw. I tend toward constipation at the slightest hint of stress. Recently on the *Huberman Lab* podcast, Professor Andrew Huberman and I were speculating about whether constipation should be a new vital sign, along with pulse, temperature, blood pressure, and breathing rate. Transit time for food from one end (mouth) to the other (anus) is an important reflection of stress load. I've been around high-stress environments for so long (e.g., the emergency room, operating room, or bedside attempting to resuscitate a patient who just died) that my bodily reaction to stress doesn't register with me until very late in the process. Until recently, I didn't notice how upset and dysregulated I was until I was pretty far gone, way out of my healthy range of function. I struggle to tell that I'm breathing shallowly, or holding my breath, or sitting too long, until I'm quite stressed and angry.

I was taught to contain my bodily sensations, and frankly, my wild animalness, in the service of thinking cogently and articulating my thoughts. This is what we are taught in grade school: to sit still, be quiet, and learn, regardless of what the body prefers. I'm not saying it's a bad thing—it got me through college, graduate school, medical school, internship, residency, and a busy career (picture a brain attached to a mouth and legs). But the default pattern meant that my body acquiesced to the demands of my mind.

Not anymore.

I have learned that there is a rich depth of communication occurring between our inner and outer worlds. And trust me, you do not want to give this up. We all must learn the language spoken by the body, even though for many of us, it's not a language that we easily understand or speak. We may try to listen only to perceive the regions that ache or are not functioning the way they once did—the stiffness in the low back, or the knee that throbs with use. We may even have developed parts that protect ourselves from feeling the pain of past bodily violations.

But what if instead we turned to our body with a sense of wonder and reverence for its mystery? You may not be able to name all the glorious biochemical reactions that are occurring in your body as you read this sentence, but I assure you they are happening on your behalf, whether you are aware of them or not.

The body is magnificent; we simply need to learn to pay attention to it.

From Dissociation to Integration

To learn the language of our bodies so that we can begin to listen, we must confront the dissociation between body and mind, which has been normalized for so many of us. What exactly is dissociation? You could think of it as tuning out, getting lost in thought, or potentially even self-abandonment. I am not in this case referring to mental illness, such as dissociative identity disorder (previously called multiple personality disorder, like in the book *Sybil*, which I read as a kid with fascination and horror), but rather a pause or break in how your mind tunes in to your body.

Dissociation is a coping strategy and a common result of trauma, much more common than I ever realized, despite practicing as a physician for years. But dissociation as a coping mechanism can have a cost. What helped me cope in childhood to distress—and may have allowed me to succeed spectacularly in school—now makes me numb out and interrupts my awareness and tracking of people who I love. It took me a few dozen years to recognize the ongoing price of my disembodiment and dissociation—specifically, workaholism, not showing up emotionally for my family, and burnout.

There's no current pill that can fix dissociation.[4] And traditional therapy alone is typically not enough to overcome dissociation either. Many of us go to standard talk therapy, which engages what medicine calls "exteroception": the focus of attention on the external world. Exteroception activates the CEO of the brain, the prefrontal cortex. As I described in the last chapter, psychotherapy got me highly skilled at focusing my attention externally and describing my experience of trauma in stories, but it didn't resolve my trauma. It reinforced exteroception but skipped interoception—the ability to sense the internal state of the body. This kind of awareness relies on other parts of the brain, including the insula (the part that integrates body awareness, sensations, feelings, and emotions) and the posterior cingulate gyrus (a hub in the brain that's involved in the default mode network and integrates internally directed thought, awareness, and memory). Interoception is not easy for people who've still got trauma embedded in their system.

It's taken years of practice for me to tune in to my body intelligence. It's required learning how to ground myself in yoga, meditation, and mindfulness; discovering how to reengage my senses; becoming an exerciser who now loves regular movement; trying somatic-based therapy; and making the effort to be more kind about the slow process of reintegration in the body. Now, after years of work, I can finally notice when and where I hold tightness (i.e., jaw, neck, shoulders; trapezius, psoas, and quadratus lumborum muscles; hamstrings, feet) and then take steps to release it. I've learned how to listen to what the body knows about why it holds on to tension and stress, and what it might take to feel safe and relaxed. I have tried a lot of techniques along the way.

We can read about embodiment or write about it, but most of us need to close our eyes to tune in to it—we need to practice the skill to go inside and truly feel internal sensation without interference from the mind or ego. Body awareness gets you deep into the present moment of what is true for you, right now. Coming home to your body and fully inhabiting it requires a new level of self-awareness.

Now we can allow the body to have its time . . . to speak, to command, to make its parts heard.

Body Scan

As I consider ways in this chapter to support your embodiment, I'd like to begin by offering a mindfulness exercise called the *body scan*.

A body scan is a mindfulness-based practice that involves scanning your body for sensations, like tingling, pain, tightness, heat, coolness, itching, buzzing, nausea, fatigue, or anything out of the ordinary. Most mindfulness-based stress reduction—which I think of as mindfulness-based *suffering* reduction—begins with a body scan, noticing without judgment each part of your body, either foot to crown or the other direction. Maybe you find places where you store tightness/distress/trauma, which for me includes the jaw and hips, particularly the psoas, known as the muscle of the soul. Where do you store toxic stress?

Below I've included a simple guided body scan, in case you haven't tried it before or if it's been a while.

SCIENCE: More than seventy-six citations in the scientific literature document the benefits of a mindfulness-based body scan. A few highlights of the effects of a ten-minute body scan:

- Provides most people with a pleasant, tingling sensation on the skin characteristic of a relaxing, flow-like state[5]
- Contributes to better emotional regulation, correlated with beneficial changes on brain scans[6]
- In healthy adults, can improve the processing of distressing memories, similar to techniques with a trained therapist[7]
- Enhances mindfulness based on a review of fourteen studies[8]
- When combined with mindful breathing, lessens symptoms of PTSD and depression in veterans[9]
- In subjects with chronic pain, significantly reduces pain-related distress and pain interfering with social connections[10]
- Reduces burnout in health-care workers[11]
- Improves interoception—your awareness of your internal state—when performed daily for eight weeks[12]
- May reduce misperceptions of physical symptoms in persons with medically unexplained symptoms and enhance decision-making[13]
- In experienced female subjects, significantly decreases diastolic blood pressure; in males, increases cardiac output during meditation[14]

Participants in the mindfulness groups experienced significant decreases in PTSD and depression symptom severity and increases in mindfulness, whereas the control groups did not.

HOW TO DO A BODY SCAN: Allow approximately ten minutes or more. Sit comfortably or lie down in a relaxed position. Take a deep breath—in through the nose and out through the mouth. Close your eyes. Start with one of your feet. Notice how the foot feels right now, and any sensations of comfort or discomfort, with a nonjudgmental stance. When you feel ready, move to the next adjacent body part—for example, from your left foot to your left ankle. Continue to the rest of the leg, then move to the other leg, then move to the belly. Keep tuning in to various body parts, finishing with the crown of the head.

Check how easy or difficult it is to slow down, turn attention away from your usual experience, and feel into your body. Body scan increases body awareness, helping you move toward body sensations, querying them, not ignoring or steamrolling over them.

If you would like to be guided through a body scan meditation, check the Resources chapter or search YouTube.

Breathwork

Breathwork has also helped me find my way back to my body. As journalist James Nestor describes in his book *Breath*, we need to reclaim the breath rather than rely on autopilot. When optimized, the breath is "a force, a medicine, and a mechanism" for gaining an almost superhuman power.[15]

Reclaiming the breath is a project we will begin in this chapter, keeping in mind that the optimal breathing rate, as Nestor defines (and as I have experienced and written previously), is about 5.5 breaths per minute, aiming for a 5.5-second inhale and 5.5-second exhale.

Subtle Energetic Body . . . Is It Real?

I studied the physical body in anatomy class in my first year at Harvard Medical School, but it wasn't until my last year, in 1994, that I learned about the human energy field. I took a monthlong seminar taught by Harvard professors David Eisenberg, MD, and Ted Kaptchuk, OMD. We reviewed the scientific basis of unconventional or unorthodox medicine, which had gained some acceptance at Harvard due to David's shocking research documenting that one in three Americans turns to complementary and alternative medicine for health benefits, at a substantial cost of $13.7 billion in 1990, most of which was paid out of pocket.[16] His paper, published in the prestigious *New England Journal of*

Medicine, woke up the conventional medical system to the reality that even if there wasn't yet a scientific basis for unconventional care, including the study of the human energy field, Americans were flocking to alternative providers for their health problems.

Later, in my thirties, I became a certified yoga teacher and learned more about the concept of the *subtle energetic body*—the presumed invisible location of potential healing, according to ancient systems. The subtle energetic body is a network of the physical, energetic, and spiritual elements of health and well-being. It consists of three components: meridians, chakras, and aura.

- **MERIDIANS** are pathways for energy within tissues that run along both sides of the body, usually in connective tissue.

HOLOTROPIC BREATHWORK®

Holotropic states are a special group of nonordinary states of consciousness. Holotropic Breathwork® was first coined by psychiatrist Stanislav Grof.[17] The word "holotropic" means "moving toward wholeness" (from the Greek *holos* or "whole" and *trepein* or "moving in the direction of something").

Process: Holotropic Breathwork® is a type of breathing practice that consists of accelerated breathing combined with evocative music in a special set and setting. Lying on a mat with eyes closed, each individual uses their own breath and music in the room to enter a nonordinary state of consciousness by utilizing a voluntary and prolonged hyperventilation procedure. It was developed to induce nonordinary consciousness during the decades that psychedelics were sent underground by legal systems throughout the world, except in Switzerland. The induced state activates the "natural inner healing process of the individual's psyche, bringing the seeker a particular set of internal experiences." With inner healing intelligence guiding the process, the experience is unique to each person and their particular setting.[18]

Roles: Holotropic Breathwork® is usually experienced in groups, although individual sessions are possible. Within the groups, people work in pairs and alternate in the roles of "breather" and "sitter."[19]

Science: Hyperventilation leads to substantial changes in the nervous system, including lessening of avoidance behaviors and enhancing therapeutic progress in ongoing psychotherapy.[20] Another study suggested that four sessions of Holotropic Breathwork® can induce beneficial temperament changes,

- **CHAKRAS** means "wheel" in Sanskrit and refers to spinning whirlpools of energy that exist in all of us but aren't seen with the ordinary human eye. However, they can apparently be "seen, felt, and sensed with intuition."[21]
- **AURA** refers to the unseen energy field that surrounds living organisms, an emanation that is an essential part of the being. Barbara Brennan, a former NASA physicist, writes that the aura consists of seven layers, each associated with a chakra (the first layer of the aura is associated with the first chakra, etc.).[22]

Is there science to support the map of subtle energy? I haven't found much. Some believe that a few of the chakras correlate with endocrine

which may decrease interpersonal problems, reduce specific undesirable traits such as being overly accommodating or needy or hostile, and increase self-awareness.[23] Holotropic Breathwork® might be useful in treatment of common psychiatric conditions such as anxiety and depressive disorders.

Why You May Want to Try It: Stan Grof described Holotropic Breathwork® as a portal to utilize the intrinsic healing potential of nonordinary states of consciousness.[24] He detailed experiences and transformations that occur not just in the usual biographical dimension (birth to present moment) but in the transpersonal dimensions of the psyche. When I first practiced Holotropic Breathwork®, I didn't go back in time to relive my conception, time in the uterus, or birth experience, but the nagging headache I had at the start of my session completely resolved. I felt better, brighter, and more grounded after Holotropic Breathwork® and have practiced it, alone or in a group, at least once per week for the past two years. Next steps: I recommend working with a certified facilitator with current professional development in the Grof Transpersonal Training (GTT) method. Only practitioners certified through GTT are allowed to practice using the term "Holotropic Breathwork®," so you may see other individuals teaching a similar type of breathwork that is not officially Holotropic Breathwork®. For the highest-quality teacher, I recommend working with a Holotropic Breathwork®–certified facilitator only. Go to http://www.holotropic.com/ to learn more and to find a certified facilitator.

organs, like the testes or ovaries; the heart chakra (fourth) with the thymus gland; and the throat chakra (fifth) with the thyroid. Others posit that chakras correlate with specific nerve bundles and other internal organs. While there are no data that I've found to support these claims, lack of proof is not proof against. We lack methods to detect chakra or auric energy, if it exists. Part of the problem is that each chakra doesn't work in isolation; researchers like to isolate cells and organs to test them in the lab, and that's not easy to accomplish with the chakra system. One article published in a peer-reviewed journal describes chakras as "energy transducers for subtle energy . . . a healing energy that anyone can perceive and utilize. It is a crucial, but often missing, component in health care."[25]

You don't need to believe in meridians, chakras, and auras to benefit from the concepts in this book. You can lightly hold these concepts and imagine that spiritual energy arises from the subtle energetic body and influences the physical body bidirectionally, if that works for you.

Wrap-Up

Over my career, I've noticed a renaissance in how we think about the individual body—it is no longer thought to exist in isolation. And what I've discovered as I wind my way back to full integration is that the body has a way of knowing what the mind does not have access to—in Hakomi terms, the body is "the royal road to the core unconscious."[26] If your body is keeping score of all the slights and traumas you've experienced, as we discussed in previous chapters, your physical symptoms might make it tough for you to hold a vision for your life that pulls you forward. But when the body is comfortable, safe, stable, and well nourished, you then have a greater capacity to reach your highest potential. On a practical level, body awareness can provide clear direction for your body type, age, and level of fitness that you need for all kinds of nourishment.

Using the practices prescribed in this chapter and upcoming chapters, I've begun to find my way back home to my body. Now I utilize my body not just as a vehicle for my mind, but as a shining intelligence that tells me whether I am on track with how I am in the world. I use signals from my body, such as areas of discomfort or subtle sensation or loss of function, to assess inspiration, discernment, and need for more self-care. I ritualize daily practices to clear the channel so that I can provide balanced attention to mind, body, and spirit.

Trust me. Once you tether your mind and spirit back to your body, and you feel whole again . . . there's no going back.

CHAPTER 7

Testing

What if disease is not, in fact, a fixed entity but
a dynamic process expressive of real lives in concrete situations?
What new (or old) pathways to healing, unthinkable within
the prevailing medical view, might follow from such a
paradigmatic shift in perspective?

—GABOR MATÉ, MD, *THE MYTH OF NORMAL*

You might imagine, or wish for, a test that tells you definitively if your nagging fatigue, joint pain, rash, hair loss, or brain fog are autoimmune in origin. But the truth is autoimmunity is mysterious. Symptoms of your body attacking itself are vague, shifting, and often nuanced—and therefore diagnosis is vague, shifting, and rarely black and white. While you're unlikely to get a simple yes/no response about whether you have autoimmune disease, in this chapter we'll explore the best way to test if autoimmunity is at play, or in even more cases, if pre-disease may be lurking in your blood, stool, and urine tests. You don't need to know all the details in this chapter; ultimately, you will rely on a relationship with a wise clinician who will work with you to review your symptoms, perform tests, complete a physical exam, and hopefully arrive at an accurate diagnosis.

Kristina, Age Forty-Two

You met Kristina briefly in chapter 1. Her story is common in my practice, and I'm sharing it again in greater detail because it demonstrates the way that conventional medicine approaches diagnosis, and sometimes fails to see the subtleties or to consider the root causes.

As you may recall, Kristina came to me at age forty-two as she faced a massive betrayal. Despite what she believed was a happy marriage, her husband left her for her friend and business partner and hid it from her. Kristina discovered their infidelity on his phone.

While Kristina was well supported by a vibrant spiritual practice, the trauma landed a major blow to her PINE network, leaving her puffy, unwell, and seeking answers. She described extreme fatigue and dipping energy in the evening. Mood swings became her norm, and she felt easily overwhelmed. While she noted a lack of focus and motivation, her elbows, knees, and ankles ached as never before. Her appetite was diminished. Her heretofore regular menstrual cycle came more frequently, every twenty-three to twenty-five days.

There is no single test that can diagnose all one hundred types of autoimmune disease, but Kristina's nurse practitioner began with a few blood tests.[1] Kristina's blood showed high levels of inflammation: not the beneficial type that heals our wounds, but the unresolved and poorly regulated type. Her complete blood count (her neutrophil-to-lymphocyte ratio) was nearly 3 and as high as 5.7 in the previous few years; (normal is less than 1). Her erythrocyte sedimentation rate (a measure of the rate at which red blood cells in anticoagulated blood descend in a standardized tube over an hour) was elevated—her level was 33 and normal is considered 0–20.

Her nurse practitioner next ordered C-reactive protein (another blood test of inflammation) and rheumatoid factor, a protein that immune cells make against tissues, causing autoimmune attack of the joint lining and usually arthritis, such as in the knee or elbow. Both tests were elevated far above normal levels. When combined with symptoms of rheumatoid arthritis and physical exam showing joint damage, high rheumatoid factor can confirm a diagnosis. However, what makes diagnosis tricky is that rheumatoid factor can also be positive when you do not have rheumatoid arthritis. It may be positive in other autoimmune conditions, viral infections, bacterial infections parasitic infections, cancer . . . the list goes on.

Her nurse practitioner referred her to a specialist in rheumatology to make a diagnosis, but it was nearly six months before Kristina could be seen. Ultimately, she saw a Stanford rheumatologist who hammered her with questions via video. Exactly which joints hurt? Precisely how long, and was the timing in the morning or later in the day? He told her he was certain that she had rheumatoid arthritis and ordered an ultrasound to document joint destruction. He recommended a medication to suppress her immune system.

She wasn't convinced. Kristina, whom I had known from attending her yoga retreats, came to me hoping to feel better again, to heal, and to use the testing to guide us. She said to me, "I am ready to feel vibrant and healthy again and commit to a plan for healing. The past two years have taken a major toll on my health, and I am needing some answers and solutions to get back to thriving."

You see, beyond the long wait for a specialist, conventional medicine has difficulty with uncertainty and may be overreliant on medication, as we uncovered in chapter 5. You are often told to adjust your lifestyle to *live with disease*, instead of collaborating on a different approach: to adjust lifestyle with a particular focus on how to resolve or reverse disease. Ultimately, adjusting lifestyle and addressing trauma may save you time, cost, and years lost due to disability.

While Kristina's case and the diagnosis of rheumatoid arthritis sets her apart, in this chapter we will explore the spectrum of diagnostic testing and certainty, what it may tell you and what it doesn't, and how it can vary depending on where you are in your transition from health to pre-disease (like me, with a positive antibody to my nuclei in my cells) to disease (like Kristina). Our goal is help you determine where you personally may be on the spectrum.

Symptom Checklist

Autoimmunity can affect a wide range of organ systems. Symptoms depend on which part of the body is being attacked, but there are a few telltale signs of autoimmunity, both the classic and common autoimmune diseases (type 1 diabetes, multiple sclerosis, celiac, psoriasis, Hashimoto's thyroiditis, etc.) and the conditions that are more newly considered to be part of the autoimmune continuum (irritable bowel syndrome, coronary heart disease, migraine, endometriosis, etc.). What you see, feel, and notice in your body—your *phenotype*—depends upon your exposure to triggers on the involved organs, tissues, and systems; your genetic vulnerability and how that interacts with your environment; and where you are located in your physiological or pathophysiological gradient.

Keep in mind that there are distinct genetic and environmental factors to consider, yet also shared mechanisms between separate autoimmune disease. In the years leading up to autoimmune disease, your body becomes reactive against your normal tissue. The first thing people notice is that the immune system is activated; the result may be low-grade inflammation,[2] which may register simply as an ambiguous sense of being unwell, tired, mentally or physically slower than usual, or foggy. This is the start of the autoimmune process, and it may take years for the disease to become fully expressed.

Check any of the symptoms below that you are currently experiencing or have noted in the past six months.

- ☑ **MUSCLE AND/OR JOINT PAIN.** Like Kristina, you may experience joint pain: achy, swollen, stiff, and tight joints, even with light activity. Exercise became more difficult as the body makes proteins that attack muscles and joints, reducing function.
- ☐ **MUSCLE WEAKNESS.** You might notice weakness in skeletal muscles that gets worse after activity and gets better with rest. It can affect big muscles like arms and legs, or little muscles, like those involved in breathing or controlling sphincters. In this case, the immune system attacks healthy muscle, leading to inflammation, swelling, pain, and ultimately, loss of function, and weakness. Also known as myositis or myopathy.
- ☐ **FATIGUE.** Typically, you wake up tired and feel like you have to push through your day. You may self-medicate with caffeine, and it just doesn't help, and long term may affect nourishing sleep and deplete you of necessary micronutrients like magnesium and B vitamins. Can progress to overwhelming and chronic fatigue.
- ☐ **INFLAMMATION.** Sometimes inflammation is obvious, like a knee that is red, swollen, hot, and tender, or a red and scaly rash. Other times inflammation may be more subtle, causing fluid retention, bloating, or

puffiness. Most clinicians check specific blood tests for inflammation, as described later in the chapter.

☐ **BRAIN FOG.** People vary in how they describe brain fog—some say it's a feeling of their brain slowing down; others describe it as difficulty focusing or concentrating. You may also notice memory changes or confusion or a decline in your normal brain function.

☐ **HEADACHE.** Sometimes considered another neurological manifestation of autoimmune disease, headache may be considered a reflection on inflammation in the brain, leading to tissue destruction and decreased blood flow.

☐ **DIZZINESS/LIGHT-HEADEDNESS.** Occasionally, people experience dizziness or light-headedness when their immune system attacks their inner ear and causes vertigo. Inflammation from other autoimmune conditions, such as lupus, can cause dizziness too. Some people have anemia or low blood count related to autoimmune disease, which can make them light-headed due to poor delivery of oxygenated blood to their tissues.

☐ **TEMPERATURE SENSITIVITY** reflects difficulty with the physiological or behavioral response to changing temperatures. You might feel more cold than other people, or more hot, and have difficulty regulating your temperature. This is common in multiple sclerosis and autoimmune thyroid disease, such as Hashimoto's thyroiditis and Graves' disease.

☐ **INTERMITTENT LOW-GRADE FEVERS OR NIGHT SWEATS.** When we see a person's body temperature higher than normal (usually 98.6 degrees Fahrenheit), we consider the possibility of infections, stress, and some medications, as well as autoimmune disease. Typically the range is 98.7 to 100.4 degrees Fahrenheit, or 37.05 to 38.0 degrees Celsius. Night sweats are a common symptom of autoimmune disease and sometimes hidden infection.

☐ **NEUROPATHY.** Occasionally we see autoimmune attack of nerves in the periphery, such as the legs or arms, or of the gut, causing nausea, anorexia, difficulty swallowing, constipation, or diarrhea. Examples are Guillain-Barré syndrome (GBS), Sjögren's syndrome, lupus, and rheumatoid arthritis.

☐ **LOSS OF APPETITE.** Sometimes this symptom is related to autoimmune attack of the gut, but sometimes it's a consequence of inflammation elsewhere, such as in Kristina's experience with rheumatoid arthritis.

☐ **GUT ISSUES**, such as acid reflux, nausea, bloating, cramping or other types of pain, loose stool or diarrhea, bloody stool, and constipation. Symptoms vary depending on which part of the gut is affected, from the stomach to the small and large intestines.

☐ **SKIN REACTIONS**, which can include a wide range of symptoms from dry eyes to dry mouth, hair loss, dry skin, rashes.

☐ **SWOLLEN GLANDS.** When your immune system is out of balance, you may notice swelling of the lymph nodes, such as in the neck, armpits, groin, under the jaw, and behind the ears. Usually with autoimmune disease, the swelling is in multiple locations in the body.

☑ **ANXIETY AND DEPRESSION.** While there's not a single cause of anxiety or depression in autoimmune disease, some believe it may be related to the increased inflammation and/or a consequence of stress or trauma. It's not always clear which came first, yet autoimmune disease can adversely affect mental health.

☐ **VISUAL CHANGES.** Sometimes autoimmune disease can cause floaters in the eye, inflammation that may trigger blurry vision or swelling, dry eyes, or double vision. You may also have difficulty with night vision or seeing colors.

☐ **WEIGHT GAIN OR LOSS.** Some folks with autoimmune disease gain weight because of the reduced physical activity and inflammation, or as a side effect of medication. Other folks may notice unexpected weight loss such as with a diagnosis of type 1 diabetes; they will urinate excessively due to lack of insulin and difficulty utilizing calories.

☐ **IRREGULAR OR RAPID HEARTBEAT.** Certain autoimmune conditions, such as lupus or sarcoidosis, may affect heart rhythm.

INTERPRETATION. Given the wide-ranging symptoms that can cluster in the hundred-plus known autoimmune diseases, it's difficult to interpret your symptoms without a clinician's expert opinion. Diagnosis depends on which body part is being attacked by your immune system. If you have three or more symptoms, I recommend starting with your primary care practitioner. If you have additional symptoms, you will likely need to see a specialist, such as a rheumatologist, endocrinologist, or gastroenterologist, for further diagnosis. They can help you sort through your genetic risk and environmental factors and chart a course for your personal health.

Beyond checking for these symptoms, you will want to assess the severity of the symptoms that you have, how long you've had them, whether the symptoms are affecting your quality of life, what seems to trigger your symptoms, the role any medications or supplements might be playing in causing or alleviating your symptoms, what else makes the symptoms worse, and if any autoimmune conditions run in your family.

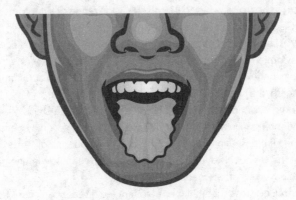

Additionally, you will want to discuss the consequences of autoimmune disease with your clinician, such as the heightened risk of coronary heart disease, leading to problems with your blood vessels, blood pressure, cholesterol levels, and coronary arteries of the heart.

Physical Exam

When examining a patient who may have autoimmune disease, clinicians are looking for any abnormalities in the skin, joints, lungs and breathing, heart, nervous system, and endocrine system. This helps us evaluate and confirm symptoms, before we layer on an assessment of biomarkers.

In my physical exam, I start with a general look at someone: their eye contact and the quality of their eyes. Then I move on to the mouth because your oral cavity is often the first place that autoimmune disease manifests.[3] Here are a few of the signs that I look for in each patient:

- Scalloped tongue, which occurs due to swelling or inflammation of the tongue. Can also be an indicator of missing nutrients, such as B vitamins and iron, or smoking.
- Midline fissuring, which is a deep groove down the middle of the tongue (on the top surface) and serves an indicator of an immune system out of balance. It reflects activation of the gut-associated lymphoid tissue (GALT) and is a sign that

your immune system (70 to 80 percent of which is housed in the gut) is overreacting. The tongue can be a window into what is happening in the GALT. Some people describe increased sensitivity of the tongue and discomfort.

I'm not an internist or rheumatologist, so I defer a complete exam to a patient's primary care doctor. Still, I perform a basic neurological exam looking for signs of neuroinflammation, like painful eye movements, changes in vision, spasticity, and changes in mental status. I check the musculoskeletal body, looking for symmetry in size, function, and any areas of weakness. I check the skin, looking for hives, rashes, plaques, or other indicators of autoimmunity. If a patient has breast implants or reconstruction after breast cancer, I'm checking for signs of breast implant illness, such as brain fog, joint pain, dry eyes, hair loss, rashes, and other concerns.[4]

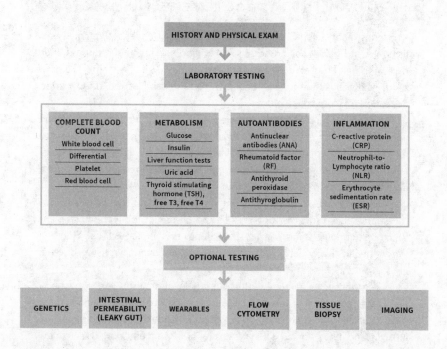

Blood Testing

When we suspect autoimmune disease, we start with a basic panel of blood tests that include the following:

- **COMPLETE BLOOD COUNT** with differential (i.e., what type of white blood cells you have and how many, the size of red blood cells and their shape)
- **METABOLISM**, including liver function and glucose
- **AUTOANTIBODIES** such as the nonspecific test for antinuclear antibodies (ANA) and/or rheumatoid factor. In Hashimoto's, may include antithyroid peroxidase and antithyroglobulin.
- **INFLAMMATION.** At a minimum, high-sensitivity C-reactive protein, sometimes erythrocyte sedimentation count (as described earlier in Kristina's story)

ANTINUCLEAR ANTIBODIES WENT UP THEN DOWN

My dentist, Mary Ellen Chalmers, DDS, is a visionary leader in functional dentistry. When I began seeing her, she asked about autoimmune disease and I explained that I had an elevated ANA test. She asked if I had metal fillings as a kid. I did: four of them. She nodded wisely. Then she looked at my tongue. Scalloped edges. Midline groove.

When I first discovered my elevated ANA test, I figured my gut/immune network was a hot mess and in need of rehabilitation. That was not news to me given my other hormonal issues that I've documented in previous books. I didn't freak because I know now to view tests as guideposts and clues, not a deterministic prison sentence.

Generally ANA is threshold, a line in the sand that those of us with autoimmunity may cross. A positive ANA can be associated with multiple autoimmune conditions including systemic lupus erythematous (SLE), Sjögren's syndrome, scleroderma, polymyositis, and mixed connective tissue disease, among others.

The good news is that even though my level of ANA was high when I first measured it in 2017, it is now negative. I've been on a path of finding the most nourishing way to heal my PINE system with healthy food and regulating lifestyle, and it has worked. I'll share several of those methods in the next few chapters.

BASIC BLOOD PANEL FOR AUTOIMMUNITY

These are the standard tests that I run for autoimmune disease:

- Complete blood count (CBC) with differential
- Metabolism: liver function tests and fasting glucose
- Autoantibodies: antinuclear antibodies (ANA) screen and rheumatoid factor. Sometimes I will check for cyclic citrullinated peptide (CCP) antibodies (another type of immune system protein called an autoantibody).
- Inflammation: high-sensitivity C-reactive protein and erythrocyte sedimentation rate (ESR)

ADVANCED BLOOD TEST TO SCREEN FOR AUTOIMMUNE DISEASE

- TSH, free T3
- Thyroid peroxidase antibodies
- Antithyroglobulin antibodies
- Rheumatoid factor
- Anti-CCP
- Celiac testing (anti-TTG, etc.)
- Anti-dsDNA
- Anti-RNP
- Anti-Smith (or anti-Sm)
- Anti-Sjögren's SSA and SSB
- Anti-scleroderma or anti-Scl-70
- Anti-cardiolipin
- Cytokines such as IL-1b, IL-6, IL-8, and TNF, are also altered in preclinical RA individuals
- Lymphocyte map using flow cytometry
- Wearables, such as continuous glucose monitoring and heart rate variability testing
- Tissue biopsy
- Imaging

If your blood contains several of these antibodies or we measure high amounts, autoimmune disease is more likely.

FUNCTIONAL FACTORS THAT LOWER THE THRESHOLD FOR IMMUNE IMBALANCE

- Abnormal HPA—dysfunctional patterns of the hypothalamic-pituitary-adrenal (HPA) axis, such as a low cortisol awakening response, a flat diurnal pattern (i.e., it doesn't go up in the morning and decline in the afternoon)
- Elevated levels of heavy metals
- Infection
- Viruses
- Bacterial imbalances, such as a predominance of a type of bacteria associated with autoimmunity in the gut flora
- Parasites
- Lyme
- Mold/biotoxin illness
- Leaky gut (increased intestinal permeability)
- Food intolerances
- Imbalanced omega-3 fatty acid pathways, leading to poor resolution of inflammation
- Cytokines associated with 5-HETE, such as IL-1b, IL-6, IL-8, and TNF, are also altered in preclinical RA individuals
- Genetic
- Poor digestion, absorption, and diversity of the gut flora

COVID and Autoimmunity: A Case Study of Self-Sabotage?

A new wrinkle in the COVID phenomenon began in spring of 2020, when it became clear that some people were not recovering quickly or easily from the acute infection. We were just a few months into the pandemic, and as is emblematic of our time, patients with lingering symptoms found each other on social media, and the terms "long COVID" and "long-haul COVID" grew traction as more people were affected and not finding answers.

What's going on? Coronavirus disease 2019 (COVID-19), which is caused by severe acute respiratory syndrome coronavirus 2 (SARS-CoV-2), has considerable overlap with autoimmune disease: joint pain, muscle pain, fatigue, dry mouth, rashes. When clinicians investigate further, we see blood clotting, inflammation of muscle (myositis), inflammation of heart muscle (myocarditis), joint inflammation (arthritis), inflammation of blood vessels (vasculitis), and inflammation of the brain (encephalitis). When you put this picture together with the volume of patients who have seemingly recovered from COVID but have persistent symptoms, it's not a stretch to imagine that the chronic inflammation of long COVID may be considered autoimmune with potentially long-term consequences. Currently, the Centers for Disease Control and Prevention has published that 40 percent of US adults have reported infection with COVID, and nearly one in five of them persist in experiencing symptoms of long COVID.[5] Overall, that's one in thirteen adults in the United States, or 7.5 percent, with long COVID, defined as symptoms that continue three or more months after contracting the virus (assuming the symptoms did not exist prior to COVID infection).

Curiously, eighteen months into the pandemic, research began to document that about half of the people hospitalized with COVID-19 had antibodies in their blood that could cross-react with their body's own proteins and tissues—was our blood mistakenly attacking our own tissues after getting infected with the virus?

The research team was led by doctors at Stanford, University of Pennsylvania, and Philipps-University Marburg in Germany, and they published their results in *Nature Communications*.[6] When they compared the autoantibodies of the admitted patients with COVID to controls, only 15 percent of controls had the autoantibodies.

Which autoantibodies? Several are described in this chapter: first, they measured antinuclear antibodies, and seeing such strikingly high rates of positive levels, they next measured double-stranded DNA (dsDNA), myeloperoxidase (MPO), and proteinase 3 (PR3) antibodies. The results confirmed what had been found previously by one of the study authors when autoantibodies and antiphospholipid antibodies were examined in subjects with a positive serology (a blood test) for SARS-CoV-2.[7] Finally, the team made a massive array of fifty-three different autoantibodies for various conditions (scleroderma, myositis, lupus, Sjögren's syndrome, mixed connective tissue diseases, gut and endocrine autoimmune disorders, and others).

It would follow that patients with long COVID would be more likely to have autoimmune symptoms and positive autoantibodies, and that is indeed the case. In a study of 106 people who were diagnosed with COVID and had their blood checked three, six, and twelve months after diagnosis, 41 percent had positive autoantibodies compared to low rates in controls.[8] Approximately 20 to 30 percent of the COVID group had blood tests indicating chronic inflammation in addition to auto-antibodies, and these were the patients who struggled the most with chronic fatigue and shortness of breath. Other studies have confirmed that autoantibodies are associated with longer duration of symptoms af-ter COVID infection.[9] COVID is common, and the potential autoim-mune component is adding massive volume to the number of us that may be affected by autoimmune illness.

Then again, we are in the learning-to-crawl stage in our understand-ing of the autoimmune theory of COVID. If the science continues to

GRADIENT OF RESILIENCY

Just like there's a gradient from health to autoimmunity, a gradient exists from low to high resilience affecting the PINE network. Some of my clients have high resilience, particularly professional athletes and executives. I test the heart rate variability (HRV, a measure of stress resiliency) of a National Basketball Association player and can't quite believe their metrics, that such exquisite states of being are possible, with HRV in the hundreds on the regular. They have their challenges, like short sleep on game days away from home, increased intesti-nal permeability and imbalanced gut flora from all of the high-intensity training and games, enormous expectations and television cameras documenting their every move (including the mistakes), and the trauma of bodies smashing into one another, but they are in the upper 0.01 percent of human performance.

Then there are the rest of us, people like me, who fly from San Francisco to New York, have one glass of wine, and HRV dips so low, it seems barely detectable. I wonder if I'm alive and how I'm able to function. Low HRV per-sists for ten days, until I get back to my protected environment at home, daily spiritual practice, organic food, people I adore, and no alcohol. Besides my stress resiliency, elevated ANA, and antibodies against gluten, I don't perform a lot of immune testing because I know my PINE is a work in progress, and I prefer to think of it as an unfolding story and less as a potentially fixed state of low resilience.

Nevertheless, when you are searching for answers and labels, it may be helpful to recognize that some of us have low resiliency centered around one support the theory, SARS-CoV-2 would join a list of many other infectious triggers of autoimmunity, including Epstein-Barr virus (EBV), a trigger for lupus and Sjögren's for some,[10] and influenza, which may be associated with a heightened risk of type 1 diabetes,[11] though the topic is still debated.[12]

Genetic Risk Factors for Autoimmunity

You can inherit an increased risk of autoimmune disease, though genes are only part of the equation. It bears repeating that autoimmune disease stems from a perfect storm of genes, environment, and the immune system: genetic predisposition gets triggered by the environment, and

aspect of the PINE system (mental health, immunity, nervous system, hormones), and some of us have low resiliency around more than one. Either you were born into the tendency for low resiliency, such as in offspring of the survivors of the Holocaust, or you developed it over time, or both. Then this position of resiliency becomes relevant when you encounter a stress test, like a preterm birth, death of a loved one, loss of a marriage, betrayal, moving parents to assisted living, major hormonal changes (pregnancy, postpartum, perimenopause, menopause), mononucleosis, COVID infection, or even a SARS-CoV-2 vaccination. In my experience, those of us with lower resiliency are more likely to have residual effects across multiple organ systems when confronted with stressors.

In my opinion, resiliency is fluid. It can improve and worsen with time. Kristina, after her betrayal, likely dipped below a threshold of resiliency and it triggered her joint pain, fatigue, and mood swings as she walked through her pain, disconnection, grief, and sadness. Now, a few years later, she is brimming with health. After that scary meeting with the Stanford rheumatologist who was so certain that she had rheumatoid arthritis, Kristina finally went to get an ultrasound of her joints about six months later. As her practitioner explained, "I don't think you have rheumatoid arthritis! I just see signs of overuse of your tendons, not destruction of your joints. You're a yoga teacher who's been teaching two to three classes every day for years. Go see a physical therapist, not a rheumatologist."

the result is an immune system that starts attacking your normal cells and tissues. While there are both distinct genetic and environmental risk factors that together trigger autoimmune pathways, pre-disease, and disease, we are still in the early stages of understanding how DNA impacts your risk of autoimmunity. Experts estimate that we have identified only about 15 percent of the genetic factors involved and how they affect inflammation pathways.[13] Still, specific autoimmune diseases like type 1 diabetes show a strong genetic association in identical twin studies, whereas others, like rheumatoid arthritis and scleroderma, show a weak genetic association.[14]

Most autoimmune disease is polygenic, meaning that the genetic risk comes from the interplay of numerous genes. It's rare that autoimmune disease is monogenic, that is, caused by a mutation in a single gene.[15]

Nearly fifty years ago, the part of the genome called the human leukocyte antigen (HLA) region was the first place we looked for the autoimmune blueprint. HLA is the part of the DNA that makes a molecule found on the surface of most cells of the body, called an antigen. Human leukocyte antigens on various cells interact with the immune system so that it can identify which cells belong in your body and which don't. The problem is that the HLA can get wonky, leading to cases of mistaken identity and immune system attack on healthy, normal cells.

The autoimmune diseases with the strongest genetic component include rheumatoid arthritis, systemic lupus erythematosus (SLE, or lupus), multiple sclerosis, and type 1 diabetes—and as a result, we see clusters of these chronic conditions in families and greater risk in first-degree relatives.[16]

Additionally, several of these diseases driven genetically can be grouped together based on HLA, including rheumatoid arthritis together with lupus, and multiple sclerosis together with type 1 diabetes. The risk is pronounced in certain genes in the HLA class. If you inherit a specific vulnerability in the HLA class, it can predispose to up to a sixfold greater risk for rheumatoid arthritis. For lupus, a type of vulnerability in HLA-DRB1 is associated with a two- to threefold greater risk of the disease in whites but not consistently in Blacks. When we look to autoimmune disease in the thyroid gland, a specific HLA gene is associated with Graves' disease but not Hashimoto's autoimmune thyroiditis.[17]

Other genes are involved too and may mediate the cross talk between genes, environment, and the immune system. While the list is long, non-HLA genetic factors include single nucleotide polymorphisms (SNPs, pronounced "snips") in immune genes, regulating immune cells or the products they make, leading to a potential predisposition to autoimmunity. However, your genetic code does not tell you if you will develop autoimmune disease; rather, it can inform us about your potential assets and vulnerabilities so that we might be able to work around them with lifestyle management, such as how you eat, move, think, sleep, and navigate toxic stress.

The Autoimmune Pattern in the Microbiota and Microbiome

Doctors aren't supposed to have favorite patients, but Larry Smarr, PhD, is uniquely fun, wise, and lovable. His remarkable career as an astrophysicist culminated at the University of California San Diego as one of the world's most famous leaders in applied computer engineering. He has data on over one hundred blood and stool biomarkers to track his health over the past few decades in one of the longest and most comprehensive time series of any person I've known. He leverages his knowledge to optimize health, directed a surgery that he needed on his gut in 2016, and put his autoimmune disease in remission, earning the moniker "Transparent Larry." He has taught me so much about the human body and how to rethink the way that medicine approaches health and disease.[18]

You might think that an autoimmune diagnosis like rheumatoid arthritis, multiple sclerosis, lupus, or type 1 diabetes has nothing to do with the gut, but that's incorrect. While the immune system is attacking tissues outside of the gut in these conditions, they all show distinct patterns of the gut microbiota compared to healthy control. These patterns, or compositions, of gut microbiota influence the autoimmune response and disease outcome.[19] The change in microbes sometimes changes the function of the immune system, and perhaps even the broader psycho-immuno-neuro-endocrine system.

Professor Smarr diagnosed himself with an autoimmune condition known as Crohn's disease, well before he had definitive symptoms. Crohn's is characterized by autoimmune attack of the tissues in the digestive tract, which can cause belly pain, diarrhea, fatigue, weight loss, and malnutrition. When diagnosed with Crohn's disease, Larry dove into experiment mode with his inputs and outputs, tracking what he eats and drinks and the qualities of his blood, stool, urine, and saliva.

After he had a nine-centimeter segment of his colon removed due to a severe stricture that he found on a three-dimensional MRI that he developed, he architected a stunning turnaround. He began drinking a daily smoothie of more than fifty different fruits and vegetables, based on the benefits to the microbiome found by his colleague Rob Knight, PhD, and his team involved in the Human Gut Project.[20] Within months and now years, he evolved to become a different Larry with a unique microbiome signature and has been free of symptoms of Crohn's disease for the past several years. His results are well-documented in the scientific literature.[21]

Larry founded the California Institute for Telecommunications and Information Technology, or Calit2, a UC San Diego/UC Irvine partnership. In Calit2's advanced visualization laboratories, you can see Larry's charts of all the changes occurring in his body, from his microbiome to his lab work to his three-dimensional imaging of his inner ecosystem.

We have known for more than a decade that the bugs in your body and their DNA (known as the microbiome) have a symbiotic relationship with our humanness, including risk of autoimmune disease. Bugs have the capacity to affect many aspects of function, including behavior, immunity, and metabolism.[22] In autoimmune thyroid disease, a pattern of increased microflora richness is seen in Hashimoto's thyroiditis, and decreased richness in Graves' disease.[23] (Note that richness and evenness are two components of diversity.[24] Generally, people with low bacterial richness tend to have more body fat, insulin resistance, abnormal lipid profiles, and inflammation compared to people with high bacterial richness.) Both groups had decreased beneficial bacteria, such as *Bifidobacterium* and *Lactobacillus*, and increased levels of harmful microbiota, like *Bacteroides fragilis*. For patients with lupus, the change in the ratio of two bacteria, *Firmicutes* to *Bacteroidetes*, may relate to development of the disease, though we are still a long way from being able to describe a specific pattern with autoimmune disease overall. Still, some patterns stand out, such as a loss of diversity and how that might relate to dysregulation of the immune system, in part mediated by microbial population.[25]

Can we then take a person with autoimmune disease and optimize their gut flora and function with healthier food, prebiotics, probiotics, exercise, vitamin D, and maybe even fecal transplantation? We don't know, but research is now being performed in earnest to try to answer these questions and offer people with autoimmune disease greater hope of remission, and maybe even a cure someday. Food may be the most important lever, as we found in Professor Smarr. In my medical practice, we use food-based recommendations and supplements first to optimize the gut flora and immune conversation, and limited research supports this approach.[26]

Areas of Uncertainty:
From Rhupus to Family History

As much as my clients love to hear universal truths about their experience in their bodies, autoimmunity offers remarkably few. While there are many shared pathways in the gradual development of autoimmune disease, as you shift from health to pre-disease to disease, you'd expect people to have specific groupings of disease.

In a previous chapter, we covered the increasing prevalence of ANA in our blood. People with rheumatoid arthritis might show positive ANA, and lupus and type 1 diabetes patients may show a positive rheumatoid factor or anti-citrullinated protein antibodies.[27]

Rheumatoid arthritis and lupus can occur in the same person, nicknamed "rhupus," but it's rare.[28] I have one patient with celiac, Hashimoto's thyroiditis, and multiple sclerosis, but that's one out of a denominator of maybe thirty thousand patients that I've seen over my career.

If autoimmune disease runs in your family, you may be at greater risk but not always for the same autoimmune disease! Genetic vulnerability may have opposing effects, such as with multiple sclerosis and type 1 diabetes,[29] or shared effects, such as with type 1 diabetes and rheumatoid arthritis.[30]

Even more uncertainty exists with the emerging overlap of COVID infection and autoimmunity. We need more peer-reviewed investigation and care to tease out the mystery that surrounds this complex chronic condition.

Wrap-Up

Beth is a forty-five-year-old mother of three living in Boulder, Colorado. She has intermittent symptoms of fatigue, muscle pain, and night sweats. Her ANA is positive, and while she has seen many specialists, including a rheumatologist, gastroenterologist, and endocrinologist, it's unclear what her diagnosis might be. Her primary care doctor noted multiple tender points on muscles, joints, and tendons that caused stabbing pain, and told her that she has fibromyalgia. Her rheumatologist refers to her condition as a "mixed connective tissue disorder, not otherwise specified." Lacking clarity about a diagnosis makes managing the symptoms difficult. She just doesn't know what she is dealing with. She has some days that leave her completely wiped out and unable to leave her bed, and other days she feels more energetic and able to see her coaching clients, but the vast space in between those experiences creates unpredictability and difficulty pursuing a career or even showing up in a consistent way for her husband and children.

Sometimes the struggle to get tested and diagnosed, or even the uncertainty of life with autoimmune illness, can leave you traumatized. I want to gently remind you that you are whole already. You happen to have a few symptoms that we may want to investigate further and address together.

Don't settle for the rote message to take a pill and be on your way. As my friend and colleague neurologist David Perlmutter reminds me, inflammation, the cornerstone of autoimmunity, can threaten decision-making, and I'd add maybe even your sense of sovereignty. If you are feeling unsure about all of the testing we've covered in this chapter, lean into a collaborative clinician about how to find the right path for you. Beware that the system can be dismissive, and sometimes gaslight your experience. If you think "gaslighting" is too extreme a term, in my survey of five thousand patients in 2022, I found that 84 percent had been gaslit about their symptoms by a physician.

Living with autoimmunity is complicated. A clear diagnosis can help provide certainty yet brings its own set of complex and serious questions about the course of illness and how to conduct one's life. Although we lack a cure for autoimmune disease, there are many treatments that have shown promise, as we will explore in the next few chapters, including specific ways of avoiding food triggers, resolving toxic stress, and providing the body with more restorative sleep.

CHAPTER 8

Nutrition Protocol

Scientists discovered that the diet triggers a death-and-life process for cells that appears critical for the body's repair.

—VALTER LONGO, PHD[1]

I f you have autoimmunity, you've probably heard a physician or nutritionist tell you that you can eat your way back to health. But it is true? Can we then take a person with autoimmune disease and optimize their health with food? Larry's experience suggests that food may be the most important lever.

In my medical practice, we use food-based recommendations and supplements first to optimize the gut flora and immune conversation, and limited research supports this approach.[2] We can heal autoimmunity by reducing or eliminating triggers, and sealing the gaps in the gut. You can potentially accomplish both with your food.

But I can tell you that the simple question of which food is best to heal autoimmunity is complicated.

Which Way of Eating Is Best for You?

Short answer: We don't know. It depends.

Scientists have studied individual autoimmune diseases in isolation; for example, the diets that contribute the best to improved function in rheumatoid arthritis are elimination diets, Mediterranean, and plant-based.[3] In multiple sclerosis, no single dietary pattern has proven to be effective in large randomized trials to reduce the number of relapses or enhancing lesions, though pilot studies on various diets, including modified Paleolithic (Wahls protocol), gluten-free, Mediterranean, low saturated fat (Swank), low fat vegan (McDougall), intermittent fasting, and intermittent calorie restriction (fasting mimicking diet), hold promise for lowering fatigue and enhancing mood and quality of life.[4] In my practice, I have found that multiple answers can be correct, and often what works for one patient doesn't work for another. And what works for most people may not work for you.

Even if you have a general sense of the type of diet that is healthiest for you, you might feel less clear when it comes to eating wheat, sugar, or potatoes, or confused about which nutrients might help to improve the immune system, such as vitamins A, B6, B9, B12, and D, prebiotics, probiotics, green tea, lipoic acid, sometimes selenium such as in Hashimoto's, and omega-3 fat. There are several published studies on how these nutrients induce particular cells of the immune system called T regulatory cells, which promote tolerance and suppress inflammation, autoimmunity, and allergy.[5]

Sometimes you know that a food makeover is needed because you have gut symptoms, like heartburn, gas, bloating, or pain. Maybe you have diarrhea or constipation, or a combination of the two. However, in my experience seeing patients, many of my clients do not feel that they have any gut symptoms, but when we look carefully at their stool test, we find that there are serious issues occurring in the gut that may or may not be related to their autoimmune disease.

Whether you have gut symptoms or not, if you have autoimmunity, research shows that an anti-inflammatory diet is a critical contributor to overall health. To reduce the inflammation caused by diet, many functional medicine clinicians recommend a strict elimination diet.

The Elimination Diet

In this section, I will cover the basic elimination diet that I follow myself and teach to my patients so that you can see if you are reacting to any of these trigger foods, or others that may irritate your immune system.

You may have heard of the Autoimmune Protocol, popularized by Sarah Ballantyne, PhD, and Terry Wahls, MD, and tested in inflammatory bowel disease, such as ulcerative colitis and Crohn's disease, and Hashimoto's thyroiditis.[6] This is an elimination diet.

The basic principle of this kind of diet is that when you remove the food-based triggers that may be contributing to your autoimmune condition, you will likely experience major improvements in your symptoms. Many of my patients even experience remission of their autoimmune disease.

Lauren is an attorney, with an ACE score of three, who woke up from sleep at age twenty-two with both hands clenched tightly closed into fists. She had just completed her first year of law school. With growing alarm, she realized her hands were stuck. Prying open each of her fingers, the pain took her breath away. A rheumatologist injected steroids between each finger to help her function.

Fast-forward to now, and Lauren has three autoimmune diseases, known in medical circles as "multiple autoimmune syndrome," which occurs in 25 percent of patients. She is rheumatoid factor negative, and her rheumatologist has diagnosed her with inflammatory arthritis; chilblains (an autoimmune condition known as cutaneous lupus erythematosus, which affects the capillary beds of the skin, usually hands or feet, resulting in redness, itching, inflammation, and potentially blisters); and Hashimoto's thyroiditis. She takes hydroxychloroquine for her arthritis and, for her thyroid, a combination of levothyroxine (T4) and liothyronine.

Most of her life, Lauren struggled with gut symptoms of reflux, indigestion, gas, and pain. A local integrative doctor ordered a food sensitivity test and it showed that she had leaky gut and was mounting an immune response against several foods, including dairy, gluten, and egg. She cut out these foods for several months as part of a gut rehab program and her autoimmune symptoms vastly improved.

Like Lauren, before I knew better, I ate wheat, sugar, dairy, processed foods, nightshades, and genetically modified foods. I washed it down with alcohol nearly every night. I binged on stress, probably related to my history of trauma and a high set point for cortisol. I suspect that all were causing increased intestinal permeability. My immune system was reacting to these foods because my leaky gut was letting reactive foods get through the tight junctions of my intestinal cells and triggering the immune system immediately below the surface. When I got rid of these foods, many of my symptoms, like mood swings, joint pain, fatigue, and chronic inflammation, disappeared within a few days.

Certain foods, like the ones that were triggering Lauren's immune reactions, and I suspect my own, increase inflammation, may aggravate autoimmune disease, and may need to be avoided or minimized.

Let's take gluten as an example. Gluten is a protein in wheat, barley, kamut, and spelt. (The protein portion of gluten is called gliadin.) Concentrations of gluten have increased in our food supply, which has led to higher rates of food reactions in the past few decades. Gluten is difficult to digest, and when gliadin breaches the barrier of the gut and gets in the bloodstream, it triggers an alarm in the immune system.

Imagine one hundred people eat a slice of bread containing gluten. Approximately seven of the one hundred may have a reaction, such as abdominal pain, bloating, heartburn, reflux, and diarrhea. Out of those seven people, one person may have celiac, and the other people will likely have gluten intolerance, also known as non-celiac gluten sensitivity (NCGS). Celiac is more severe, putting people at risk for anemia, fatigue, headaches, joint pain, psychiatric disorders, and low vitamin D and B12, and can lead to malnourishment. For celiacs, gluten must be completely avoided for the rest of their life. People with NCGS, like Lauren and me, can limit or eliminate gluten to reduce symptoms.

Celiac is an autoimmune attack of the small intestine, triggered when genetically susceptible people consume gluten and have increased intestinal permeability.[7] It affects about 0.5 to 2 percent of the population. The autoimmune attack depends on a complicated immune response, resulting in antibodies that attack the small intestine.

When antibodies in the blood attack gluten, they may also react against normal tissues too, like your thyroid, in what's known as molecular mimicry. The net result is that if you have autoimmune thyroid disease such as Hashimoto's thyroiditis or Graves' disease, and you eat a bowl of pasta containing gluten, your immune system may attack your thyroid in a case of mistaken identity. Overall, there is a strong association between autoimmune thyroid disease and gluten intolerance,[8] and all people with autoimmune thyroid disease should be screened for gluten intolerance (and if you have gluten intolerance, check for thyroid problems!).[9]

Another way that food can trigger inflammation and autoimmunity is by forming immune complexes. Think of these like a pair of wrestlers fighting for power; gluten (gliadin) and the antibodies that bind to gluten create a complex that travels through the bloodstream. The wrestling immune complex, gliadin and its antibody, courses through the body with destruction in its wake, while the rest of the body looks on, not sure what to do.[10] Normally, the immune system can remove the immune complexes from the blood, but when the volume is too high, it's more than it can handle. The complexes land in various organs, creating more inflammation and damage, and ultimately autoimmune consequences, like painful, puffy joints. However, cutting out gluten removes the immune complexes.

While gluten isn't the root cause of all autoimmune disease, it contributes to autoimmunity in many conditions. Besides gluten, other important contributors to autoimmunity, both positive and negative, are fiber, fat, and nutrients.

If the right diet can ease symptoms and help you heal from autoimmune disease, how does that work?

Several studies have looked at the elimination diet in rheumatoid arthritis (RA). Overall when you consider the randomized, double-blind, placebo-controlled trials, approximately 30 to 40 percent of RA patients improve on an elimination diet.[11] People with RA who are superresponders may be able to discontinue pharmaceuticals, and research shows that some of them may be in remission for more than a decade. If you have RA and start an elimination diet, the response occurs within three to five days, and most studies evaluated a total duration of ten to twenty-one days. Not surprisingly, benefits disappear when you resume a normal diet. An elimination diet seems to shift the gut flora in a beneficial direction, leading to improved immune function, though we are still trying to understand the precise mechanism and changes seen across the people who try it and are successful.

How to Do the Elimination Diet

To follow a basic elimination diet, cut out all of the potential triggers for three weeks to three months. If you have significant gut symptoms, you may need to be at the longer end of the spectrum.

Phase 1: Elimination. You will want to be off all of these ingredients and foods for a minimum of twenty-one days.

- Dairy
- Gluten
- Alcohol
- Grains
- Eggs
- Sugars (especially high-fructose corn syrup)
- Red and processed meat
- Processed and ultraprocessed foods
- Nightshade vegetables (potatoes, tomatoes, eggplants, et al.)
- Caffeine
- Peanuts (not a nut, it's a legume, and has increased chance of triggering immune reactions)
- Nuts
- Seeds
- Other common triggers: industrial seed oils, food additives, artificial sweeteners, emulsifiers, food thickeners

While the list may feel exhaustive, I find that some people can begin with cutting out a few of the worst offending foods, like dairy and gluten, and feel improvements in symptoms. Other people need the full-scope elimination diet, meaning that they detect which ingredients are poorly tolerated and relieve food allergies or intolerances by removing all of the suspected foods from their diet listed above.

If it is overwhelming to perform all eliminations at once, cut a few at a time. However, keep off of all of them at least twenty-one days, because it takes a minimum of twenty-one days for the immune system to become less trigger-happy and reactive. Wait until you cross the three-week mark before you decide if it is working. An elimination diet is not an ongoing lifestyle choice; it is a short-term diagnostic test. We are testing whether it helps your pre-autoimmune or autoimmune symptoms. After eliminating 100 percent of these ingredients for a minimum of three weeks (or longer—up to three months—if you've been struggling with autoimmune disease for more than one year), you will start to reintroduce one food at a time and observe for three days how you respond digestively and more system-wide.

You may wonder what is left to eat. Focus on vegetables, fruits, healthy fats, and SMASH fish (salmon, mackerel, anchovies, sardines, and herring—the safest, most nutrient-rich fish, which are least likely to be high in mercury and tend to be the healthiest). You'll want to rotate the foods you eat, like our hunter-gather ancestors used to do.

ALL DISEASE BEGINS IN THE (LEAKY) GUT . . .

More than half of my patients have some degree of increased intestinal permeability, or leaky gut, including most of my athletes and all of my clients with autoimmunity. Unfortunately, despite more than a decade of robust science of how increased permeability is at the root of autoimmunity from venerated institutions like Harvard, the University of Chicago, and the Mayo Clinic,[12] medical institutions are slow to agree that it is an important issue to address in the care of patients with autoimmunity. Our physicians need to heed Alessio Fasano, MD, who first published about increased intestinal permeability and its connection to celiac and other autoimmune diseases back in 2006. He is a professor of pediatrics at Harvard Medical School, professor of nutrition at Harvard T.H. Chan School of Public Health, chair of Pediatric Gastroenterology and Nutrition at Mass General for Children, and director of the Mucosal Immunology and Biology Research Center at Massachusetts General Hospital. One of my favorite article titles is "All Disease Begins in the (Leaky) Gut: Role of Zonulin-Mediated Gut Permeability in the Pathogenesis of Some Chronic Inflammatory Diseases."[13]

Why is increased intestinal permeability so common? It's our diet, alcohol consumption, chronic stress, toxin exposure such as to glyphosate, and imbalanced microbes in the gut. These lifestyle factors disrupt the delicate tight junctions in the gut, and we now know that dozens of proteins play a role in keeping tight junctions functioning properly. When they are working, they allow nutrients to pass through the junction and enter the bloodstream below, and they keep out unwanted factors like bacteria and toxins. If you have leaky gut, symptoms may be gut-related, including gastric ulcers, irritable bowel syndrome, small intestinal bacterial overgrowth, or diarrhea, or they may seem unrelated to the gut—for instance, joint pain, arthritis, allergies, respiratory infections, chronic immune response syndrome (CIRS), fatty liver, chronic fatigue, obesity, thyroid disorders, and autoimmune disease (celiac, Hashimoto's thyroiditis, inflammatory bowel disease like Crohn's and ulcerative colitis, lupus, multiple sclerosis, and type 1 diabetes).

To help repair your gut barrier, make sure you are getting nutrients like vitamins A, B, D, zinc, and healthy fats; additional supplements may be called for too.[14] For many of my patients, I recommend consuming bone broth–based soups and powders containing L-glutamine, which may help seal leaky gut.

They ate nuts, seeds, berries, fish, and animals, and they ate seasonally, so they varied their diet based on the time of year. (Rotating the foods in your diet helps to avoid the risk of an immune or allergic reaction to the food.) Today, for example, I ate leftover shredded chicken scrambled with chopped chard, served with gluten-free avocado toast, for breakfast. Lunch was a Cobb salad, hold the cheese. Dinner was salmon with an artichoke, and sauteed purple cabbage with bok choy.

You might be wondering about good swaps for the foods you cannot have, the ones that are likely triggering your immune system. For getting off of caffeine, reduce coffee intake by switching to half decaf for a few days, then herbal tea. If bread is your emotional support, change to gluten-free bread (and read my story about emotional eating in chapter 11). If cheese is your favorite, consider the new cheeses (see Resources—they are now scrumptious). If sugar is your Kryptonite, go with monk fruit or stevia while on the elimination diet. Check out the Whole30 books and community for additional ideas.

An elimination diet is not rocket science, but clear instructions can be helpful, so if there is not sufficient information provided here, consider checking out the Autoimmune Protocol developed and refined by Sarah Ballantyne, PhD.

Phase 2: Reintroduction. After three weeks at a minimum, start to add one ingredient back at a time and test how the body responds, which is known as the "provocation" phase.

To get the full benefit of your experience, reintroduce one food at a time very thoughtfully and methodically. Just because we call this an elimination diet, don't be fooled: this reintroduction and testing stage is of the utmost importance. In some ways, the reintroduction is the opposite of elimination, but it's also more purposeful in that it tells you which foods might be triggering your immune system. It's also where I see the greatest mistakes. I see clients who decide "I'm tired of this process, I'll just eat pizza"—and they have gluten plus dairy plus nightshades all in one sitting and then don't know which one of those three is triggering their joint pain or other symptom. So please engage fully in a purposeful reintroduction as it will make the previous three weeks pay off.

If you notice that your symptoms are improved by the end of the first three weeks, you likely have an immune reaction to one of the foods you are testing. Now we get to determine which food or ingredients are the trigger. It can take up to seventy-two hours to see delayed hypersensitivities, so you must give yourself a minimum of three days to assess your response to each food. How to do it? Take a small dose of the food or ingredient you are testing. Have it at the same time each day, usually breakfast, for three days in a row. For example, if you are testing dairy, you might have a half cup of yogurt made from cow milk at breakfast each morning, together with allowed foods (berries, or another fruit). Then track your symptoms, like energy, mood, brain fog, hives, rashes, joint discomfort, swelling, or gut issues. If you have a reaction, continue to eliminate that food, then move on to test the next food or ingredient, such as gluten.

Troubleshooting: Some of my patients tell me that they previously tried an elimination diet and it didn't help their symptoms, and usually I find that they didn't eliminate all of the ingredients listed above or they added too many of the ingredients back at the same time in the provocation phase, thereby losing the opportunity to gather useful information about their unique biology and triggers. During the first week, you may notice that you feel withdrawal for certain foods, including gluten and dairy, due to their opioid-like (morphine-like) effects. Typically withdrawal symptoms abate by the second week and you may notice better sleep, energy, focus, pain, and general function.

Nutritional Modulation

As noted above, the elimination diet is a diagnostic tool. But what principles should you keep in mind when you eat for the long term? There are four main areas to address via nutritional modulation when you have an autoimmune disease: nutritional gaps, poor digestion, toxic backlog, and blood sugar spikes.

1. **NUTRITIONAL GAPS.** When I take care of a patient with autoimmune disease, or a pre-autoimmune condition, I look first for nutritional insufficiencies and deficiencies because they are common. They occur from eating the typical Western diet, inflammation, celiac, imbalanced gut microbes, and food sensitivities. Micronutrients are essential

dietary elements—vitamins and minerals—that you need for physiological function and optimal health, like B vitamins and magnesium. The amount you need varies depending on life stage—you'll need more as an adolescent and in pregnancy and usually less as you age. Micronutrients are not usually produced in the body and must be obtained from the diet (the one exception is vitamin D, which your body makes when exposed to natural sunlight). Macronutrients are the dietary elements that we need in higher quantities to obtain energy: fat, protein, and carbohydrates. Both micronutrients and macronutrients can be inadequate for your needs.

2. **POOR DIGESTION.** When your digestive tract is not doing its job—which is to process food, fuel your cells, and eliminate waste—you may feel symptoms such as the following, all of which are common in autoimmune disease.

   - Fatigue
   - Bloating
   - Constipation
   - Diarrhea
   - Heartburn
   - Bleeding
   - Fecal incontinence
   - Nausea
   - Abdominal pain

   Digestion is tricky to figure out, so I recommend working with a functional medicine clinician to learn how to assess and address it.[15] Most of my patients need additional functional testing, described in the notes from the Introduction, and supplements that help them digest food, such as betaine HCl and digestive enzyme.

3. **TOXIC BACKLOG.** You may wonder how toxins and autoimmunity relate to each other. We get hit by toxins as daily occurrence—makeup, skin creams, furniture, water bottles, and cleaning products in the home. Much of the toxins work to disrupt your delicate hormone balance, and

while one toxin on its own may not be enough to cause symptoms, the cocktail of many at once can be enough to cause problems with hormones and blood sugar such that increased inflammation is triggered, and in someone who is vulnerable to autoimmunity, this can sometimes be a trip wire to cause illness. I find that about half of my patients have sluggish detoxification pathways that they inherit leading to buildup of toxins in the body. These toxins get stored in fat instead of being correctly excreted in urine, stool, and sweat, so one of our first tasks together is to improve detoxification while also reducing toxic load, starting first with food and then moving on to lifestyle. Tried juicing as a way to detox? I'm not usually a fan of juice other than as an occasional treat. Eating organic foods, eating and drinking from glass containers, and limiting use of plastic can make a big difference, as can increased sweating through exercise and taking sauna.

4. **BLOOD SUGAR SPIKES.** Blood sugar problems can be common in autoimmune disease, including type 1 diabetes

---

FIBER

As the unsung hero of autoimmune recovery, fiber helps you detoxify because it binds to toxins in your gut and escorts them to the door—out of your colon and into the toilet. It can also help prevent you from reabsorbing them. When you eat foods that are rich in dietary fiber, like fruits and vegetables, the gut microbiota ferment the fiber into beneficial molecules called short-chain fatty acids, which have anti-inflammatory effects as shown in the massive study by the Women's Health Initiative (whose results on hormone replacement therapy have been revisited and partially debunked, but which still hold merit for other findings).[16]

You can count how many grams of fiber you are consuming each day either manually or with an app. Aim for 30 to 40 grams per day, but if you're way below that dose, like most people, slowly increase by no more than 5 grams per day to avoid bloating, cramping, and constipation. Our hunter-gatherer ancestors ate 50 to 100 grams of fiber per day, but our guts may struggle with that much. The types of fiber that I like best are listed in the Resources; they are powders that can be used to supplement your fiber intake from food so that you can get to the recommended dose each day.

WHAT ALCOHOL DOES TO YOUR GUT

When researching leaky gut in animals, there is an easy way to create it with near certainty: give alcohol to the animals. Chronically drinking alcohol damages the delicate cells of your gut by increasing the permeability of the intestines, leading to leaky gut. When your gut is healthy, the cells of your gut are arranged tightly together like a defensive line, creating a barrier that protects the immune system that lies beneath the surface. The barrier is meant to regulate what gets to pass through the surface and what keeps going through the tube and ultimately to be emptied as your stool. Susan Blum, MD, describes the barrier like a brick wall where the intestinal cells are the bricks and the mortar between the bricks are called tight junctions. Additionally, there's a coating of mucus on top of the intestinal cells called the mucus layer that provides additional barrier protection. However, when you lose the barrier with a leaky gut, you are more likely to develop autoimmune disease. Many things can cause leaky gut, like imbalanced microbes, toxic stress, certain medications, hard exercise particularly in athletes, chemotherapy, and viral infections—but one of the most common root causes is consuming alcohol. When you have leaky gut, you may have symptoms of constipation, gas, or bloating, even brain fog, or you may have no symptoms.

Studies in animals and humans show that most of the damage, such as erosions and bleeding, occurs in the small intestines as well as the stomach and liver. Some people think that their bowel movement after one to two glasses of wine is a good sign of lubrication, of a positive effect of alcohol on their tendency toward constipation, but that's not true. Alcohol is causing damage. However, a smaller amount of alcohol, ideally fewer than three servings per week, may be less harmful, but we don't really know. The truth is that I enjoy the first few sips of wine the most, and that's unlikely to cause leaky gut. The good news is that if you are like me and enjoy sipping wine, the intestinal lining turns over every three to five days, plus the entire mucus layer is replaced every one to two hours! So there is some forgiveness in the system as long as you don't assault it with alcohol on a daily basis.

and autoimmune thyroiditis, and likely others as well. When we look to the root cause, sometimes it is related to increased stress and perhaps underlying trauma leading to adrenal glands that produce excess cortisol. High cortisol raises blood sugar and can also trigger a greater immune response. The typical spiky blood sugar response to food can be seen in someone like me, who has a significant trauma load and stress. I eat an apple (or some other food with a substantial amount of carbohydrates), and it triggers excessive insulin release. My blood sugar rises steeply from the apple, and then crashes from the exaggerated insulin release, so that I have a big spike of glucose that goes way up and then way down. You can see these types of responses in a device like a continuous glucose monitor. In terms of what you feel, you might immediately notice symptoms like fatigue, a drop in energy, anxiety, panic, and light-headedness, but it also overtaxes the adrenal glands over time. The glucose spikes can damage blood vessels too, causing a greater risk of cardiovascular disease later in life. When you learn how to eat in a way that stabilizes blood sugar, you'll find that you feel more energy and calm.

Wrap-Up

It astounds me that what you eat and drink can be the potential cause of autoimmunity, or the most nourishing influence in terms of helping to prevent or reverse autoimmunity. The brilliant gastrointestinal system determines whether your nutrition is adding value or harming you. It's thrilling that up to fifty billion cells are shed in the intestine every day.

Astonishment aside, I realize that a strict elimination diet is a tough ask. While it's difficult to implement and maintain for twenty-one-plus days of what can feel like a sacrifice, a well-constructed elimination and provocation process will pay dividends over decades. Take your time and do it well.

While I agree that the gut is at the root of autoimmune disease, and the best way to upgrade the gut is with food, we are still a long way from knowing exactly what works best. Food isn't the only tool in your toolbox, as there are many other environmental, social, and lifestyle issues that we now know can promote chronic inflammation, potentially leading to cardiovascular disease, cancer, diabetes, chronic kidney disease, neurodegenerative disorders, and autoimmunity.[17]

Still, research from the past decade on the interface of the gut, immune system, and microbiome has greatly increased our understanding about nutritional immunomodulation. Most of my patients who put their autoimmune disease in remission are fully committed to a diverse diet in which they consume the colors of the rainbow and get regular exposure to sunlight for healthy immune function. That's where we begin in terms of turning the ship around and supporting a stronger foundation that helps them return to health.

CHAPTER 9

Sleep and Stress Protocol

Each of you is perfect the way you are . . .
and you can use a little improvement.

—SHUNRYU SUZUKI ROSHI

S leep is as close to a panacea as we have for your health. We've all noticed the miserable effects of poor sleep and lousy stress management, but science shows that it's not just short-term misery at stake. If you have autoimmune disease, sleep deprivation and high perceived stress can amplify systemic inflammation and pain sensitivity, making an already overtaxed immune system go into overdrive and potentially worsening disease. Sleep and stress also have a major impact on mental health. Dysregulated cortisol, the main stress hormone, is a risk factor for suicide, along with disrupted sleep and other factors, like childhood trauma, impaired executive function, impulsivity, family history, and epigenetic and perinatal experiences.[1]

Joanna is a forty-three-year-old physician with several diagnoses, including Ehlers-Danlos syndrome (EDS) and likely Sjögren's syndrome.[2] She had a long history of joint hypermobility, autonomic dysfunction (she has frequent fainting since childhood), and gastrointestinal dysmotility as a result. Five years ago, she also developed bruxism, involuntary and habitual clenching of her teeth during sleep.

A few years ago, Joanna's parents died abruptly and violently from a car crash; the tragic and traumatic loss was profound for Joanna at many levels. Her bruxism worsened and she developed instability on the left side of her jaw that caused popping and clicking and made it hard for her to chew on that side. Botox injections didn't help much. Was trauma linked to her development of autoimmunity and bruxism? We don't know for certain, but the timing is suggestive. As we will describe later in the chapter, she began addressing her trauma in a novel way with psychedelic medicine, which had a powerful impact on sleep and subsequently resolving her bruxism and improving her overall functioning.

Bruxism can be a sign of poor sleep and too much stress. In the majority of my autoimmune clients, sleep and stress are huge influences, both in positive and negative directions. When sleep is sound and stress is well managed, they light up the grid of the nervous system. The biological benevolence of sleep spreads from there to the immune and endocrine systems.

Sleep and stress are deeply encoded, often from childhood, and may require significant intention and compassion to change. Improving either is not a one-and-done campaign, nor was Joanna's treatment approach. Any trauma or neuroses driving autoimmune tendencies won't disappear overnight, but you can start watching them with curiosity, witnessing them in a way that provides more options for possible improvement. For example, you might ruminate at bedtime, saying to yourself (with compassion), "Oh, there I go again. There's that thing I do . . ." Are you deferring the dog walk until noon, missing the morning sun? Watching an extra episode of a television show that keeps you glued to the screen for an hour later than you planned? Pay attention to these behaviors.

I've written previously about sleep and stress and ways to mitigate damage when either or both are off. In this chapter, I've focused on the latest data and trends, and if you're a longtime reader, you will find new techniques that I've been working with for the past few years—solutions that truly work for my patients and me. Even if you're jaded and feel like you know everything possible about your own sleep and stress, read on. As a skeptical veteran of the sleep and stress wars, I remind myself that fresh eyes and ears are sometimes the best approach to getting these aspects of healing back on your side.

Sleep Matters

While conventional medicine tends to ignore sleep debt, I do not. Disturbed sleep affects most of my patients, from NBA players who are on the road during the season and playoffs to perimenopausal women wondering when they can expect to sleep again through the night. One-third of Americans have excessive daytime sleepiness. The average night of sleep in the United States is 6.9 hours, and what's needed is a minimum of 7 to 8.5 hours every night.

Good sleep is essential to a healthy PINE system. Sleep is the critical time when the body repairs its cells and reduces inflammation. We know that sleep and autoimmunity have bidirectional effects: sleep is disrupted by autoimmune disease, and poor sleep can make autoimmune disease worse.

Sleep is the way to prime your body for healing. While you sleep, the brain removes debris and cleanses itself, the gut repairs, and the immune system strengthens. It sets up your circadian rhythm or clock, the natural internal process that regulates not just your pineal gland in the brain, which produces melatonin, but nearly every cell of your body. That's why sleep has such a massive and broad effect on your health, and is foundational to healing from pre-autoimmunity and autoimmunity.

Yet half of people with arthritis struggle with falling asleep. More than half rate their sleep quality as poor, or not refreshing. In a national study of 4,200 people with rheumatoid arthritis, nearly two-thirds had at least one sleep disorder, such as short sleep syndrome (less than seven hours of sleep at night), restless legs syndrome, or obstructive sleep apnea, according to researchers from the University of California at San Francisco.[3] The worse the disease activity and pain, the higher the association with criteria for an abnormal sleeping pattern. It makes sense that the pain and disability of rheumatoid arthritis and other autoimmune diseases can make sleep more difficult and disrupted.

If you already have sleep problems but not autoimmune disease, take note. Sleep problems increase your risk of developing a new case of autoimmune disease. This was discovered in a study of 84,996 Taiwanese people with a non-apnea sleep disorder, compared to a control group of 84,996 urban adults.[4] In this large study over three years, there was a 47 percent greater risk of developing a new autoimmune disease in the poor sleepers, particularly lupus, rheumatoid arthritis, ankylosing spondylitis, and Sjögren's syndrome.

Sleep and Trauma

Traumatic life events can disturb your sleep-wake cycle.[5] Trauma has long been linked to a particular type of disrupted sleep that includes nightmares and hyperarousal in cases of PTSD, though I see both of these problems in people with partial PTSD too. Not surprisingly, childhood trauma can cause sleep issues in adulthood.[6] Known as parasomnia, trauma and related causes such as anxiety and depression can cause abnormal sleep patterns that may run the gamut from sleep terrors to sleepwalking, sleep-related eating disorder, and sleep paralysis.

Trauma, big *T* or little *t*, can make it difficult to sleep acutely (short term) and chronically (long term). Experts agree that out of the various sleep cycles and stages, the part of sleep that is more affected by trauma is rapid eye movement (REM) sleep. REM is pivotal to your health and well-being because it's the stage for processing emotions and storing memories, and dreams during REM are often more wild and curious. In my opinion, they often reflect the unconscious more accurately than dreams in other sleep stages.

More recently, clinicians and researchers are using a newer term known as "trauma-associated sleep disorders" (TSD), though how TSD differs from the overlapping conditions of PTSD and rapid eye movement sleep behavior disorder (RSB) is still in question.[7]

People with higher levels of post-traumatic stress and PTSD tend to have more severe and persistent sleep disorders.

Given that experiencing trauma can negatively affect sleep, the combination can erode your mental and physical health, putting you at greater risk of autoimmunity or worsening existing autoimmune disease. You may have more trouble falling asleep, awaken more during the night, and have difficulty going back to sleep. My usual pattern is that I wake up at four a.m., wide awake and hyperalert, ready for the day even though my body needs more rest. Even if you don't believe your history of trauma or toxic stress is significant, many of us have a pattern ingrained of ruminating at night. Address it! The good news is that additional effort with normalizing sleep after trauma has been shown to reduce trauma-associated memories and to make them less distressing.[8] You may find that both the sleep tips in this chapter and the stress and mindfulness tips in chapter 11 can help you regulate your sleep and heal.

How to Measure Sleep

The most accurate way to measure your sleep is with a clinical sleep study, known as polysomnography. The test involves sleeping overnight in a laboratory, where clinicians will check your brain activity and identify which stage of sleep you are in and for how long. Of course, sleeping in a lab isn't the best place for a good night of sleep. Consumer devices attempt to capture similar data but are not as accurate. Are they accurate enough? The answer is "probably."

Consumer sleep trackers are reasonably accurate at measuring total sleep time and at tracking both light sleep and rapid eye movement (REM) sleep. You can use this information to improve your sleep and start a conversation with your doctor. I like to use them for directionality, such as if your REM sleep is low, that usually means you need to go to bed earlier. If you don't have enough deep sleep, you may need to work on gut health.

I use sleep trackers with nearly all of my patients and clients. We use them to perform n-of-1 experiments and to see what's going to work best for an individual. In a recent study of six wearables, several rose to the top, and the researchers confirmed what I've seen in my medical practice: that Oura ring tends to be the best, along with the Somfit forehead device and WHOOP wristband (see Resources for additional details).[9] Most of my experience is with Oura, which has been subject to rigorous scrutiny in terms of accuracy.[10] They all make an educated guess about your sleep stage information without the brain activity data, so unless you perform polysomnography, be skeptical about the accuracy but aware of the direction your tracker may be pointing. Review your findings with your trusted health-care provider, and consider trying the lifestyle changes listed next to see if any aspect of sleep improves. If you are not ready to invest in a sleep tracker, listening to your body will give you the clues you need to decipher your quality of sleep. Journal in the morning how well rested you feel and track what routines were helpful in generating that well-rested feeling.

When I wake up in the morning, I make a pot of tea and meditate. Next I review my sleep data and ask new questions. I ask how I can be more consistent about my bedtime, with an aim to be in bed, ready for sleep, by ten p.m. I look outside and wonder how I can enjoy early morning bright light, even on a cloudy day, and bring my meditation cushion outside. I look at my calendar for the day and ask if there are schedule changes that could make sleep a higher priority, to support sleep hygiene. I query, "What are the main stressors in my life right now that may be disturbing my sleep?" I note my total sleep time, aiming for 7 to 8.5 hours, which is associated with the longest healthspan,[11] or the period of time you are free of chronic disease. If I don't get seven hours, I plan a nap that day. When I first began tracking my sleep about five years ago, my main problem was low deep sleep, usually an hour or less. Once I rehabilitated my gut following the elimination diet in the last chapter and the sleep principles in this chapter, my deep sleep is regularly one to two hours in duration—I've found that gut health is at the root of better deep sleep for me and others. REM sleep has improved too, thanks to consistent sleep hygiene—that's our goal!

Sleep Architecture

Normal sleep is organized as illustrated in the chart on page 138. At its simplest, sleep is divided into two categories, non-rapid eye movement (NREM) sleep and rapid eye movement (REM) sleep. NREM sleep is further divided into N1, N2, and N3 sleep (formerly stages 1, 2, and 3). N1 is when you close your eyes and fall asleep. N2 is when your body relaxes further. N3 is deep sleep, also known as slow-wave or delta sleep. Some consider it the most important because it's the deepest stage of sleep—it restores and heals the body and the mind is allowed to rest. The last stage of sleep is REM. Matthew Walker, PhD, an expert on sleep, calls REM sleep "informational alchemy," because we make connections and revise the mind-based web of associations as well as prune synapses to foster learning. REM can also reduce activity in the amygdala, which is the part of the brain involved in fear, anxiety, and stress, and make you feel more emotionally regulated.

You cycle through each stage in approximately ninety-minute increments. Usually the first cycle is the shortest, 70 to 100 minutes. Later cycles last 90 to 120 minutes. Early in the night, you tend to get more deep sleep whereas later cycles have more REM. A sleep tracker may help determine which part of the sleep cycle is getting short-changed and help you adjust your bedtime to best meet your own sleep needs. Getting a full seven to eight hours of sleep helps you move through each stage so you relax your body, refresh your mind, reset your immune and endocrine systems, store and consolidate memories, and emotionally regulate.

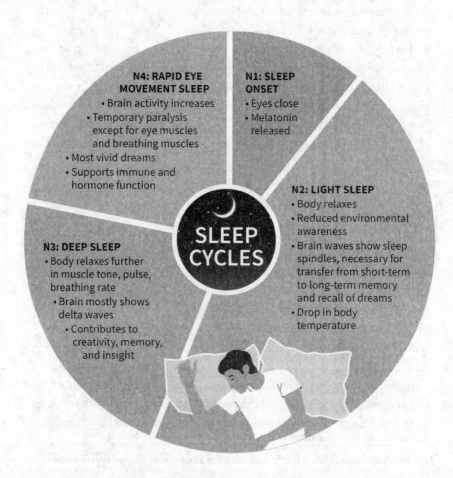

EIGHT STEPS TO BETTER SLEEP

Step 1: Measure your baseline.

Step 2: Reestablish at all costs and reinforce your circadian rhythm. Get natural sunlight first thing in the morning. Eat and drink at the right times, including the limitation of alcohol (or avoidance, since it pokes holes in your gut and makes you more likely to have autoimmune flares). Generally, I tell my patients to eat three hours before bedtime, but with autoimmune disease, digestion prior to sleep is paramount, so I recommend eating a light meal at least four hours before bedtime.

Step 3: Exercise before noon.

Step 4: Take the TV, phone, and other devices out of your bedroom. This limits blue light and will make it easier for you to go to bed on time.

Step 5: After sunset, avoid artificial light at night (i.e., break up with ALAN).

Step 6: Take sleep nutrients, like magnesium glycinate, phosphatidyl serine, or an herbal aid that contains valerian, passion flower, chamomile, and lemon balm.

Step 7: Put yourself to bed like you would a small child. I take a hot bath nearly every night, and add various elements to the bath like essential oils and Epsom salt.

Step 8: If you're still not sleeping 7 to 8.5 hours every night, consider a wearable like Oura or WHOOP.

Sleep and Stress

Healing from autoimmunity requires the cultivation of resilience not only by improving sleep, but also by reducing stress. The more you diminish the impact of toxic and traumatic stress, the less likely you will be to experience disrupted sleep.

"Stress" can be a vague term, and that makes it difficult to neutralize. You may be thinking to yourself that you already have learned everything you can about stress. I agree with you. I find more conventional approaches to stress to be a waste of time and money. For stress mitigation, I like to quantify stress at baseline so we know what we are up against and to do it in a way that is sustainable yet effective but very efficient. You can glimpse into a window of how your nervous system is functioning and your stress response in one of two ways: with a self-report test or a physiological measurement. My favorite self-report test is the Perceived Stress Scale, which you can google and track over time.[12]

For physiological measurement of stress, I like to measure cortisol and heart rate variability (HRV). I track my HRV daily with an Oura because it's the best way I have found to track my nervous system and capacity to train and perform. HRV may be the easiest way to assess your psychophysiology. It measures the amount of time that fluctuates between your heartbeats, and perhaps surprisingly, can portend health problems like cardiovascular disease, depression, and anxiety. You may hear that HRV is a measure of the balance between the sympathetic nervous system (the "on" part of the stress response system) and the parasympathetic nervous system (the "off" button). When you're under significant stress, the most common pattern is that you get high sympathetic activity and low parasympathetic activity.[13] HRV can also reflect your capacity, performance outcome, and recovery. See the Resources for my favorite ways to measure stress, including Oura Ring and WHOOP.

Toxic Stress: What to Do

When the medical system failed to help me with persistent cortisol problems, I found ways that work for me to manage my stress, and then found that most (if not all) of the solutions work for others. Know what helped me more than anything else? A fresh take on my boundaries with others and where they need to be reinforced; spending more time with friends, family, and colleagues who fill me up; and psychedelic medicine delivered in a safe environment by a knowledgeable health-care provider. Many of my clients, patients, and cases have found similar results.

I've written for the past ten years about all the things I've done. I've learned from others to wrangle stress and used that learning to develop a framework to help you discover what might work for you.

STEP 1: Measure your baseline. Either check your stress level on the Perceived Stress Scale, or invest in a wearable that checks your heart rate variability or similar metric. If using a wearable, get a solid baseline over several days of measurement and record the average value of the HRV or composite metric, for example, Oura's "Readiness" score or Garmin's "Body Battery."

STEP 2: Choose one of the stress resilience techniques listed below to try for the next four weeks:

- **MEDITATION.** While twenty minutes a day may be ideal, most of us can truly benefit and relax our nervous system starting with just five minutes once per day. Dial in the daily frequency first with the minimal effective dose, then once established, slowly increase duration.
- **MINDFULNESS.** At its simplest, mindfulness is the practice of bringing one's attention to the present-moment experience without judgment. It's an acceptance of what is. You can try a local class, watch a YouTube video, or check out the free online course mentioned in the Resources.
- **NATURE.** Get a daily dose for at least twenty minutes in order to activate the parasympathetic nervous system of "rest and digest."
- **YOGA.** Yoga's physical postures, breath control, and concentration help to create resilience. You can start with just one or two simple poses.
- **READ** a book or an inspirational ancient text.
- **SIGHING.** More specifically, *Huberman Lab*'s physiological sighing—we discussed how to do it when I was on Andrew Huberman's podcast recently.[14] Briefly, you take a max inhale through the nose, then another short nasal inhale, then full exhale to empty lungs via the mouth. Repeat for five minutes. In a clinical trial that Dr. Huberman performed at Stanford, physiological sighing was compared to box breathing and hyperventilation.[15] All had benefits, but sighing had more in the twenty-four hours after practicing.
- **WALKING A DOG, OR BEING WITH A PET.**
- **SPENDING TIME WITH FRIENDS, FAMILY, AND PEOPLE** you enjoy, whether in person or over the phone.

STEP 3: During these four weeks, perform the technique you've chosen once per day and track what happens to the metric you measured in your baseline in Step 1. Does the metric improve? How long does it take to improve? If it doesn't improve after four weeks, is there another technique that you want to try next?

Joanna's Blueprint

While Joanna sought help from experts for her dysautonomia, autoimmune, and connective tissue conditions, she also recognized that her trauma and now PTSD were playing a significant role in the symptoms she was experiencing. She sought treatment in the form of ketamine-assisted psychotherapy. After only one session of therapy augmented by intramuscular ketamine, she began sleeping again and her bruxism was barely noticeable. It was as if the anger and trauma she had been carrying were stored in her jaw, and through the ketamine journey they had been released. The result was an incredible relief.

Unfortunately, Joanna found the relief required continued treatments every two to four weeks, and this was not ideal given her busy life. It was clear, however, that the psychedelic medicine had tremendous power to alleviate the physical symptoms she had been experiencing by facilitating the processing of her trauma. She told me that it felt "like the ketamine was resetting [her] nervous system." Maybe the ketamine treatment helped to reduce the progression to full autoimmune disease.

Later, given the success—albeit temporary—of the ketamine therapy for her PTSD, Joanna attended a ceremony with ayahuasca with the hope that this medicine may provide a more permanent resolution. Indeed, this experience offered Joanna a profound healing: "I felt the medicine extracted the last stitches of PTSD bound to my soul. And as it left my body, my jaw relaxed into comfort and ease."

Wrap-Up

More than seventy years of evidence demonstrates that psychological and social factors are key to the chain of events that connect the psychosocial to immune-neurological-endocrine disturbances. And yet stress and trauma tend to be treated like an excuse to avoid looking further at why someone is experiencing an illness like autoimmunity. Even though sleep and stress initiate a series of known biochemical processes involved in the autoimmune cascade, it's as if conventional medicine just doesn't want to deal with them, or perhaps doesn't know how.

I know how, because I have struggled with stress, poor sleep, and trauma. One thing I know for sure is that as you observe the feelings surrounding sleep and stress issues, if maybe shame comes up, don't be mad at yourself. It's just what the egoic mind does. Don't overidentify with the thought, or the story; just witness it. You don't have to be tyrannized by it. My advice: take one sleep tip from this chapter and work with it consistently each day.

CHAPTER 10

Immunomodulator Protocol

We are eating hybridized and genetically modified foods full of antibiotics, hormones, pesticides, and additives that were unknown to our immune systems just a generation or two ago. The result? Our immune system becomes unable to recognize friend or foe—to distinguish between foreign molecular invaders, we truly need to protect against the foods we eat or, in some cases, our own cells. In Third World countries where hygiene is poor and infections are common, allergy and autoimmunity are rare.

—MARK HYMAN, MD, FAMILY PRACTICE PHYSICIAN AND MULTIPLE *NEW YORK TIMES* BESTSELLING AUTHOR

John was a fifty-two-year-old corporate attorney at the top of his game. He was working from five thirty a.m. to ten p.m. daily, interacting with his firm's top clients in a demanding role. One day during an especially stressful time at work, he felt a "snap" in his skull and became dizzy. In his office, he lay on the floor, unable to sit up or stand. The skin around his lips went numb. He called his physician, who was concerned about a stroke and told him to go immediately to the hospital, and he went with a friend in a cab. An MRI suggested multiple sclerosis. He was hospitalized for four days and given Solu-Medrol, a form of steroids, which is often given in autoimmune disease to quell inflammation. He was sent home on a taper of oral steroid pills and Avonex,

IMMUNOMODULATOR PROTOCOL 145

and a prescription injection of interferon beta-1a, a very strong immunomodulator used in patients with multiple sclerosis. Immunomodulators are usually a short-term way of manipulating the immune system to your benefit. John would take an interferon beta-1a injection weekly on a Thursday, and for the following thirty-six hours, he experienced flu-like symptoms akin to his immune system fighting an infection with muscle aches, fever, chills, and fatigue.

John's case reveals the strong association we often see in autoimmune disease between genetic vulnerability, leaky gut, and then an environmental trigger, like the toxic stress that he experienced at work. We can't change the genetic code. We can address leaky gut as we covered in chapter 8, and toxic stress as we covered in chapter 9, but when those are not sufficient, we can turn to immunomodulation. The good news is that there are many natural immunomodulators that you can consider short of a prescription biologic.

Your Immune System Can Sense and Cause Trouble

As you've learned in Part 1, innate immunity is the first line of the immune response that reacts to cell stressors, danger signals, and foreign ("nonself") invaders like viruses and bacteria. When you have a healthy innate immune system, it functions as both a detective and a first responder that defends the body against attack and promotes repair. The system is sophisticated, but when it works against you, as it does in autoimmunity, the solutions may not have to be as fancy as the biological immunomodulators that John was prescribed.

Diet and lifestyle medicine can create more engaged and regulated health of the innate immune system. The gut microbiota, housed in the gut and environs, are responsible for maintaining the balance between host defense and "tolerance" of the immune system. It's a two-way street: the gut microbiota help to keep the innate immunity healthy and balanced, and the innate immune system (gut-associated lymphoid tissue, innate lymphoid cells, and phagocytes—the vacuum cleaners of the immune system) likewise can affect the gut microbiota, and both are potentially influenced by food and supplements. Microbial disruption, like from taking antibiotics or even getting exposed to glyphosate from crops treated with the weed killer Roundup and other glyphosate-based herbicides (note that glyphosate is the active ingredient in Roundup), can perhaps alter the delicate innate immune response and potentially increase the risk of diseases like cancer[1] and other chronic diseases,[2] though data are mixed and the narrative is still evolving.[3] Certain autoimmune diseases may be associated with disruptions in the gut microbiota/immunity axis, particularly rheumatoid arthritis and lupus, and to a lesser extent, systemic sclerosis, Sjögren's syndrome, and antiphospholipid syndrome.[4]

I've been interested in the role of nutrition, such as the use of polyphenols and antioxidants, in creating immune health for many years. I help an NBA team use nutrients as a competitive advantage over other teams; the nutrients alter gene expression and the tendency toward inflammation and help regulate the immune system.[5]

So how do we reestablish regulation of the innate immunity in a way that may help avoid the march toward autoimmune disease? If autoimmunity requires three components—genetic predisposition, leaky gut, and environmental triggers—we can work with immunomodulators to address leaky gut and the impact of environmental triggers.

What Is Immunomodulation?

Immunomodulation is when we use an agent or lifestyle technique to modify the immune system, usually to activate or suppress immune function. Immunomodulation can be natural or synthetic, and both approaches are aimed at improving self-regulation and homeostasis in an immune system that has undergone betrayal of some form, usually autoimmune disease. John's prescription for Avonex is called a biological response modifier (BRM) in the pharmaceutical industry, and it's used to treat a variety of autoimmune diseases.[6] Other BRMs include additional agents you may have heard of, such as erythropoietins, interferons, interleukins, colony-stimulating factors, stem cell growth factors, monoclonal antibodies, tumor necrosis factor inhibitors, and vaccines.

But there are other agents in the medical bag. First, as discussed in chapter 8, a healthy diet, low in immune triggers and rich in nutrients, is fundamental to mitigate inflammation and oxidative stress.[7] Secondly, we can target the immune system with natural immunomodulators. Be-

BIOMARKERS OF THE INNATE IMMUNE RESPONSE

You can track the performance of the innate immune response with readily available tests:

- **C-reactive protein (CRP)** checks for inflammation in the body with a protein made by your liver. Normally, you have low levels of CRP, but if you experience inflammation, the liver releases more CRP into the bloodstream.
- **Erythrocyte sedimentation rate (ESR)** also checks for inflammation in the body. ESR measures how quickly red blood cells separate from a blood sample that has been treated so that the blood does not clot. When you have inflammation, the red blood cells tend to clump together, resulting in a high ESR.
- **Neutrophil-to-lymphocyte ratio (NLR).** When you draw blood from a vein and count the proportion of immune cells present as neutrophils versus lymphocytes, you can calculate the ratio between the two groups of white blood cells. Neutrophils roughly reflect the innate immune system, whereas the lymphocytes indicate the status of the adaptive immune system. Normally, the ratio is less than one. When it's higher, the client is more likely to have excess inflammation in the body.
- **Myeloperoxidase (MPO)** is a measure of an enzyme produced by neutrophiles, one of the white blood cells.[8]
- **DHEAS.** I measure DHEAS levels in all of my patients, and often find that people with low DHEA (less than one hundred) are more likely to experience autoimmunity. It's not clear that supplementing with DHEA helps in these cases because we lack randomized trials, but DHEA plays an important immunomodulatory role.[9]
- **Visual contrast sensitivity (VCS)** test measures your ability to see contrast, so it provides an indication of neurological function related to contrast sensitivity, which can be impacted by the innate immune system when it is dysregulated by mold exposure in sensitive individuals.[10]

low are a few immunomodulators, which I use regularly in my medical practice, that we will explore in this chapter to see if they are right for you. Some are oldies but goodies, like antioxidants (vitamins A, C,[11] D, and E[12]), fiber, omega-3 fatty acids,[13] curcumin, and vitamin D. Others are relatively new to the scene like mushrooms (psychedelic and nonpsychedelic), hormones, peptides, and low-dose naltrexone. Note there are areas of overlap with other molecules not mentioned here—for example, cells lining the gut and several types of immune cells show vitamin A and D receptors, and both vitamin A and D can alter the expression of tight junctions that keep the gut barrier intact and functioning appropriately.[14]

- Black cumin
- Other polyphenols: curcumin, epigallocatechin gallate, quercetin, resveratrol
- Vitamin D
- Antioxidants
- Anti-inflammatories such as omega-3s and specialized proresolving mediators
- Low-dose naltrexone
- Peptides
- Exercise
- Mushrooms, including microdosing of psychedelics

BLACK CUMIN (*NIGELLA SATIVA*). Cumin is a common spice in Northern India, Pakistan, and Iran. Black cumin is a variety of cumin used medicinally in various healing systems, including Ayurveda. In autoimmune disease, black cumin has been studied in multiple clinical trials in patients with Hashimoto's thyroiditis.[15] In forty patients with Hashimoto's thyroiditis, a randomized, placebo-controlled trial showed that treatment with black cumin for eight weeks reduced body weight by a few pounds, and lowered body mass index, thyroid stimulating hormone (TSH), and anti-thyroid peroxidase (TPO) while raising serum T3 levels.[16] The same group found that black cumin favorably changes lipid levels.[17] Limited studies, including one randomized trial, have been performed with black cumin in rheumatoid arthritis and show potential benefit.[18] Other studies have suggested a significant anti-inflammatory effect.[19] Dosage used in the trials was a daily dose of 2 grams of black cumin, milled in a grinder.

POLYPHENOLS. Polyphenols are a large family of naturally occurring and beneficial agents that you find in foods, particularly fruits and vegetables but also tea, herbs, spices, dark chocolate, and red wine (don't get too excited—alcohol is one of the surest way to cause leaky gut, so I'm not recommending it). There are over eight thousand types of polyphenols.[20] Overall, polyphenols can lower blood sugar,[21] reduce your risk of heart disease and blood clots,[22] promote healthy gut function, impact mitochondria favorably,[23] change gene expression,[24] act as antioxidants—meaning they scavenge molecules in the body known as free radicals that can damage cells and DNA[25]—and may lower the risk of autoimmune disease.[26] I'll highlight a few of the most proven polyphenols that I prescribe to support immunomodulation: curcumin, epigallocatechin gallate, quercetin, and resveratrol.

CURCUMIN. I have a food-first philosophy when healing autoimmunity, and the food that contains curcumin is turmeric root. I chop it and add it to soup bases and scrambles, which you can think of as the modern-day stir-fry.[27] Not everyone has access or time to deal with turmeric root (or the way it stains your hands and cutting board), so supplementation can sometimes be helpful. Why take curcumin? Because curcumin lowers inflammation in people with autoimmune disease (as measured with blood tests for C-reactive protein and erythrocyte sedimentation rate, described in chapter 7 on testing),[28] and it has been shown to reduce intestinal permeability.[29] The latter study is fascinating because a low dose worked so fast: in a small study of eight people with increased intestinal permeability, curcumin (500 milligrams per day for three days) was shown to normalize the function of the gut barrier. Three days! Generally, I recommend a curcumin dose of 500 to 1,000 milligrams per day.

EPIGALLOCATECHIN GALLATE (EGCG). EGCG is one of the active components of green tea. It has many health-promoting features in terms of reducing inflammation, acting as an antioxidant, and modulating the metabolic system, and recently its immune activity has been investigated. It is a well-known immunomodulator that has been shown to reduce autoimmune activity in patients with autoimmune disease.[30]

QUERCETIN. Found in many foods and plants, such as green tea, apples, berries, capers, green tea, kale, red onions, and red wine, quercetin is a plant pigment (flavonoid) that provides color. Recent research suggests that quercetin may reduce inflammation and autoimmune activity in inflammatory bowel disease, multiple sclerosis, rheumatoid arthritis, and systemic lupus erythematosus in humans or animals, as well as in allergic conditions.[31]

RESVERATROL. Derived from berries, grapes, chocolate, and other plants, resveratrol has activity in many pathways from reducing inflammation to helping guide estrogen metabolism in the right direction, which may also impact autoimmunity. First isolated in 1939, it is the subject of more than twenty thousand research papers, making it the most studied polyphenol. Unfortunately, the aggregate of the data demonstrate varying results, and significant controversy exists about whether it can affect metabolism and extend healthspan.[32] Regarding autoimmunity, resveratrol reduces inflammation and progression of autoimmune disease in animal and human studies of inflammatory bowel disease, psoriasis, rheumatoid arthritis, systemic lupus erythematosus, and type 1 diabetes.[33] Dose 500 milligrams/day for six weeks or longer.[34]

VITAMIN D. Low vitamin D levels in the body are linked to various health risks. Vitamin D regulates calcium balance in the body, but it may be the natural agent that does the most in terms of affecting the gut and modulating your immune system. It turns up or down the genes that regulate inflammation and alter the response of the immune system, and it interacts directly with immune cells involved in both innate and adaptive immunity.[35] Vitamin D is critical to the maintenance of the gut barrier, such that it's the careful filter it's meant to be, not a sieve.

Taking supplemental vitamin D reduces your risk of developing a new autoimmune disease.[36] In the VITAL clinical trial of nearly twenty-six thousand people, taking vitamin D (2,000 IU per day) with omega-3 (1,000 milligrams per day) lowered the risk of incident (new) autoimmune disease by 22 percent.[37]

What about if you already have an autoimmune disease? Will taking vitamin D help you feel better? The question hasn't been tested in clinical trials, and other research shows the data are mixed.[38]

Vitamin D is involved in both innate and adaptive immunity, and it may be a potential lever to prevent or treat autoimmune disease. How do we know that vitamin D is involved in the immune system? There are several lines of evidence: mucosal cells that make up the gut's inner lining express vitamin D receptors, so giving vitamin D can alter the expression of tight junctions that keep the gut barrier functionally intact; potentially block viral infection, such as by COVID, by interacting with the cell receptor;[39] and help to keep the absorbing fingers of your gut lining (called microvilli, located in the duodenum) longer and potentially more functional.[40] When vitamin D levels are low, animal models show that tight junctions and intestinal permeability are worse than when vitamin D levels are normal.[41] Taking vitamin D helps to repair the gut and improve symptoms, both in animal models[42] and in people with Crohn's disease, though it doesn't address all aspects of gut permeability.[43] I typically start with Vitamin D3 with Vitamin K2.

ANTIOXIDANTS. Food-based antioxidants and sometimes supplements like glutathione, N-acetyl cysteine (the precursor to glutathione), lipoic acid, vitamins C and E, beta-carotene, selenium, copper, zinc, and iron have been shown to reduce inflammation and oxidative distress and can support a healthy immune response and potentially provide protection in cases of infection.[44] The way it works is that oxidative stress, as indicated by overproduction of reactive oxygen species, may promote the onset of specific autoimmune diseases.[45] When reactive oxygen species accumulate and are not quenched by antioxidants, cells are damaged, leading to autoantigens mediated by innate immunity.[46] Several autoimmune diseases are characterized by depletion of antioxidants like vitamin C, so it makes sense that keeping levels at a healthy level may be supportive.[47] Studies of the use of antioxidants show modest benefit, and while I don't believe every single antioxidant needs to be taken, I would focus on the primary antioxidant, glutathione. You can increase levels with N-acetyl cysteine at a dose of 600 milligrams twice per day for three months, which has been shown to reduce morning stiffness and biomarkers of inflammation in rheumatoid arthritis.[48]

OMEGA-3 FATTY ACIDS AND SPECIALIZED PRORESOLVING MEDIATORS (SPMs). Omega-3 long-chain polyunsaturated fatty acids (e.g., fish oil, which is the most potent anti-inflammatory fatty acid) may improve health in people who tend toward autoimmunity. My preference is to eat omega-3s by consuming two servings or more per week of freshwater fish or shellfish to reduce chronic inflammation.[49] We evolved as human beings with a good balance between omega-3 and omega-6, yet our modern diet has led us to eat too many omega-6s, which are found in processed food and corn, soybean, grapeseed, and canola oils. Crowd out the less-healthy omega-6s with healthier omega-3s and the omega-6s that your body craves, such as from gamma-linoleic acid, evening primrose oil, and borage oil. In clinical intervention studies of people (besides the VITAL trial mentioned previously) with multiple sclerosis, psoriasis, rheumatoid arthritis, systemic lupus erythematosus, and type 1 diabetes, outcomes improved with supplemental omega-3 fatty acids.[50] Does consuming omega-3s prevent autoimmunity? We don't know for sure, but one study from Denmark showed that you can reduce your risk of rheumatoid arthritis by nearly 50 percent for each 30-gram increase in daily fatty fish consumption.[51] Doses of fish oil in most trials were approximately 2 to 4 grams (e.g., for a 2.2-gram dose, 1,350 milligrams of eicosapentaenoic acid, and 850 milligrams of docosahexaenoic acid daily).

Specialized proresolving mediators (SPMs) are a newer discovery that may help with the chronic inflammation of autoimmune disease, though randomized trials have not been performed.[52] You can take the dose listed above for omega-3s and add two to three softgels of SPMs (follow directions on the supplement bottle).

LOW-DOSE NALTREXONE (LDN). Naltrexone is a drug that we've been using in medicine for fifty-plus years to treat opioid and alcohol addictions, and in the course of treatment for addiction, we learned that lower doses can be a safe and inexpensive way to treat autoimmune disease, chronic pain, and a condition that may span both realms called fibromyalgia—people with fibromyalgia have chronic, widespread pain, tenderness, and fatigue.[53] At this point, LDN has mild to unclear efficacy with different autoimmune diseases and other conditions, including rheumatoid arthritis and multiple sclerosis, so more research is needed. [54] One study of 360 patients with rheumatoid arthritis from Norway showed that LDN reduces the need for other medications like pain medication (opioids and nonsteroidal anti-inflammatory drugs) and prescription immunomodulators like TNF-α antagonists.[55] Based on the limited evidence in Hashimoto's thyroiditis,[56] I offer LDN occasionally to my clients, particularly people who haven't responded well to conventional thyroid medications and agree to an n-of-1 experiment to see if it helps. In these circumstances, use of naltrexone is "off label," and dosage is 1 to 5 milligrams per day.

PEPTIDES. Peptide therapy for autoimmune disease seeks to rebalance the immune system via signaling the T cells and the thymus gland, which is a small organ in the chest under the sternum that makes lymphocytes. Injectable peptides such as thymosin alpha-1 may be given because the thymus gland begins to degenerate after age thirty. While there are case reports of benefits, we lack large clinical trials, so this method is considered experimental.[57]

EXERCISE. While extended periods of intense exercise training can cause immunosuppression and leaky gut, moderate exercise performed regularly tones and supports the immune system.[58] It reduces inflammation in people without autoimmunity,[59] but what about when you cross the threshold into autoimmune disease? Evidence is limited but mostly promising in rheumatoid arthritis, lupus, inflammatory bowel disease, and multiple sclerosis,[60] though one study showed a lack of benefit in myasthenia gravis. Technology may help us clarify the immunomodulatory role of exercise in autoimmune disease, such as the use of continuous glucose monitors in type 1 diabetes.[61] In rheumatoid arthritis, high-intensity interval walking for ten weeks was associated in a pilot study of twelve people with improved cardiorespiratory fitness, lower blood pressure and resting heart rate, better innate immunity biomarkers, and a decline in disease activity by 38 percent. Participants saw less swollen joints and significant reductions in inflammation as measured by blood levels of erythrocyte sedimentation rate (ESR).[62] In one study, one cycling ride reduced aggressive (cytotoxic) T cells.[63] Just one ride!

Another study of forty-five patients with myasthenia gravis, an autoimmune disease that attacks the communication between nerve and muscles, leading to unsteady walk, droopy eyelids and mouth, and difficulty swallowing, showed that a moderate-intensity home rowing program three times per week for forty minutes over three months led to no changes in quality of life.[64] We need more research on how exercise might immunomodulate autoimmune pathways.

Can Mushrooms Modulate Your Immune System?

It's been a banner year for mushrooms, and with good reason. Mycologist Paul Stamets believes that mushrooms are essential to a healthy immune system in not just people but larger ecosystems. (Yes, ecosystems or habitats have immune systems, as you may have noticed during the recent pandemic.) Immune systems decline in response to stress, exhaustion, and disease—and I've seen firsthand how taking mushrooms may support a more balanced immune system.

How does it work? There's a physiological mechanism that is still being worked out, and there is a more metaphorical mechanism. Metaphorical first: mushroom molecules, according to biologist Merlin Sheldrake, PhD, "have found themselves entangled within human life in complicated ways exactly because they confound our concepts and structures, including the most fundamental concept of all: that of ourselves. It is their ability to pull our minds into unexpected places that has caused psilocybin-producing magic mushrooms to be enveloped within the ritual and spiritual doctrines of human societies since antiquity."[65] Physiological next: mushrooms activate beneficial aspects of your immune system, including lymphocytes, macrophages, and natural killer cells.[66] We lack randomized trials showing beneficial immunomodulation with mushrooms, but investigations are underway. You'll learn more about psychedelic mushrooms in chapter 12.

Wrap-Up

Autoimmunity is a combination of cells attacking the body and over-production of antibodies against your own tissues, which galvanizes loss of immune tolerance and rogue immune responses. Immunomodulators may help, and the natural immunomodulators explored in this chapter are important tools to help regulate the immune system again and call off the self-attack. Before beginning any immunomodulators, I recommend that you work with a trusted clinician who is familiar with the agents described in this chapter and also aware of any interactions that may occur with other medications that you are taking.

CHAPTER 11

Mind-Body Therapy Protocol

It takes courage . . . to endure the sharp pains of self-discovery rather than choose to take the dull pain of unconsciousness that would last the rest of our lives.

—MARIANNE WILLIAMSON, *A RETURN TO LOVE*

Natalie is a forty-eight-year-old third grade teacher. The last few years have been particularly challenging as she's shepherded her students through the pandemic, Zoom classes, and the return to the classroom. Few of her kids are neurotypical and most have high adverse childhood experience (ACE) scores. One of her students is a girl from Guatemala who passed into the United States inside of a refrigerator truck. Another student was beaten so badly as a toddler that he required a craniotomy. Now he is neurodiverse, and occasionally lashes out at Natalie, kicking and punching her. Several parents are active drug users. Natalie is on the receiving end of the trauma behaviors. "It's nuts," she tells me. "Sometimes I don't feel safe in my own classroom, but I'm stuck. If I could do something else to make money and put food on the table, I would. Meanwhile, I'm just coping by eating comfort food and trying to get through each day, surviving from one weekend to the next."

Natalie has been teaching for twenty-five years. Previously, she would head home after work and pour herself a few glasses of wine each night to cope. Her drinking started to affect her health and marriage, and she found her way to a twelve-step program and turned her life around with their mind-body approaches. There was no cost. While twelve-step programs are not specifically designed to address trauma, it allowed Natalie to develop a relationship with a power greater than herself, establish a daily spiritual practice, and create ways of coping with toxic stress and trauma so that they don't eat at her the way they once did.

Nurses and teachers have the highest burnout rates of professional workers, probably as a result of dealing with the grind of caring for humanity up close. Natalie has noticed immunological effects from the trauma she experiences: her right knee is swollen like a cantaloupe at the time of her visit, and her orthopedic surgeon tells her that she needs platelet-rich plasma (PRP) injections. As we have detailed in previous chapters, toxic stress, shame, and guilt can trigger the PINE system to get out of whack. An added layer of self-blame causes the greatest inflammatory response.[1]

In chapter 5, we covered why traditional drugs and talk therapy aren't necessarily sufficient to resolve trauma for most people. What's often missing is the somatic component that we covered in both chapters 5 and 6. Additionally, people with significant trauma such as PTSD usually benefit from trauma-informed therapy, which involves recognizing the presence of trauma symptoms and acknowledges the role trauma is playing in a person's life.

In this chapter, we will dive into the therapies that have been effective for many people, myself included, and I'll share with you the top three techniques that my clients have found to be the most healing. While there are many other mind-body techniques to consider, some of which I've described in chapter 5, there are three that I've found astonishing: Hakomi mindfulness-based somatic therapy, Neuro Emotional Technique (NET), and the twelve-step program as developed by Alcoholics Anonymous (AA).

The Promise of Mind-Body Therapies

Mind-body therapies are a constellation of healing techniques that improve the functional relationship between the mind and body toward a particular goal, usually to induce relaxation, improve health, or create integration. Typically, daily practice is essential in order to benefit from these therapies.

In autoimmune disease, the immune system attacks healthy cells in the body by mistake and creates excess inflammation. Mind-body medicine can help you reduce inflammatory responses without the side effects shown to be associated with conventional anti-inflammatory medications like steroids, nonsteroidal anti-inflammatory drugs (NSAIDs), and immunosuppressive agents.

My friend Terry Wahls, MD, explains that we have two million biochemical processes happening in our bodies each minute, and a drug affects just one or two of them. On the other hand, lifestyle medicine, including nutrition, sleep, and mind-body therapies, can affect hundreds, even thousands, of these reactions. While a pill or injection may seem like an easier answer, they don't always activate healing as broadly and deeply as lifestyle medicine.

Why invest in mind-body therapies? First, they seem to be the most important needle mover for my clients. Second, they are fun and potentially transformative. Third, in a classic study of sixty-three patients with rheumatoid arthritis randomized to a Mindfulness Based Stress Reduction (MBSR) eight-week course followed by four-month maintenance, the MBSR group had a 35 percent reduction in psychological distress and well-being compared to a control group after six months.[2] That's a profound improvement, on par with and sometimes better than what expensive immunosuppressive medications can provide.

In this chapter, we will investigate the mind-body therapies that I have found to be the most effective for my clients with autoimmunity and trauma, including Hakomi, Neuro-Emotional Technique, and twelve-step programs. I have personally explored all of these modalities for my trauma and toxic stress and found that they all help me develop witness consciousness (the capacity to *witness* the mind, or peacefully observe its machinations, without overidentifying with it or to be distracted or disturbed by it) and allowed me to recover from disordered eating.

While some or all of the mind-body therapies may sound woo-woo, the idea is that when you are in a trauma state, it's like you are riding the advanced Class 4 or 5 rapids of a river. If you're like me, you are in fear of drowning or dying, not looking at the root cause of why you are in the rapids or how to get to safety. You are just trying to survive, to keep your head above the water. I heard this described by Michael Singer about survival, and I believe it translates well to living with trauma. The worse your response to trauma, the more you get stuck in survival mode, stuck in one rapid after another. You have to get your head above water enough to develop perspective, agency, and the ability to navigate the rapids. That's what you get with mind-body therapies—you get your head above the water, above the noise. Your consciousness extricates itself from being stuck in the process and can now watch it so you're open to more options and healing.

Recommendation #1: Hakomi (Mindfulness-Based Assisted Self-Study)

In the inimitable words of the opening line of the Hakomi guidebook, "Mindfulness has gone viral."[3] Hakomi is a method of bringing unconscious material to the surface where it can be skillfully integrated and healed in a rapid yet gentle manner. Psychologist Ron Kurtz developed Hakomi beginning in the 1970s. He was a brilliant man, knowledgeable about systems theory and steeped in the wisdom traditions of Taoism and Buddhism. He resisted calling Hakomi "therapy," preferring to consider Hakomi "assisted self-study." While it may sound like a type of sushi roll, you have to experience Hakomi yourself to understand its profundity.

"Hakomi" is a Hopi Indian word that means "How do you stand in relation to these many realms?," an ancient way of asking, "Who are you?"

I began seeing a Hakomi therapist in 2022. After decades of talk therapy, my Hakomi sessions unwound many difficult memories and toxic stress from the past. I found missing nourishment. I responded so well to Hakomi's assisted self-study and self-discovery that I signed up for the comprehensive training. Personally, I've found that it helps me rewire neural hardware and "shift these organizers of experience through the function of attention."[4] I feel happier, clearer, and more fully alive. After just a few sessions, I noticed more contentment, trust, safety, and stability, despite my relatively high adverse childhood experience (ACE) score.

The system of Hakomi is elegant and complex. Briefly, the guided self-study of Hakomi uses mindfulness to access the memory system where fundamental unconscious beliefs are encoded. Those beliefs color our perceptions and responses to life, but we can reshape them. While not specifically designed as "trauma-informed" care, trauma therapy has been developed within the Hakomi framework by practitioners such as Manuela Mischke-Reeds[5] and Pat Ogden.[6] Unless a Hakomi-certified therapist or practitioner has advanced training in trauma, referral is recommended to avoid putting clients into a state of reexperiencing trauma.

One of my teachers describes Hakomi as a method that allows one to experience nonegocentric nourishment. Ron Kurtz describes the method in this way: "Self-study is a natural part of the universal human endeavor to free ourselves from suffering, the inevitable suffering that results from ignorance of who we are and how the world hangs together."

See the Resources for more information and to find a Hakomi-certified therapist or practitioner near you.

Recommendation #2:
Neuro Emotional Technique (NET)

All of us have suffered traumatic events in our lifetimes, whether a health scare, divorce, death of a loved one, humiliation, bullying, or failing at a crucial task. Often these events resolve themselves over time, without intervention. Other times they continue to live on, weigh down your quality of life, and trap you in ways you may not realize. NET provides a way out. It's not the only way, but it's the one we have found to be most efficient and effective. NET is a holistic mind-body approach for exploring and releasing *stress-related conditions* in the body.

My chair at Thomas Jefferson University, Daniel Monti, MD, has performed several research studies on NET. In the *Journal of Cancer Survivorship*, he and his team reported that cancer survivors who had distressing events showed dramatic objective and subjective improvements after only three to five sessions of NET.[7] One of the study's outcome measurements was a brain scan using functional magnetic resonance imaging (fMRI) performed while each patient listened to a description of their distressing event. The description was based on interviews with the patient and was recorded using their own words as much as possible. This same protocol was followed before NET treatments and after NET treatments. There was a control group who went through the same protocol but did not receive any NET intervention.

The study revealed three dramatic observations.

- The brain scans demonstrated for the first time in cancer survivors the effects of the distressing event in real time in the parahippocampus part of the brain before NET treatment—the parahippocampus is one of the structures in the emotional/feeling part of the brain.
- The brain scans demonstrated dramatic resolution of a distressing cancer-related event, as reflected in the now greatly diminished activation of the parahippocampus.
- For the first time, it was observed that the cerebellum of the brain is involved with emotional regulation, as seen by changes in the communication pathways between the cerebellum and other brain structures. Previously it had only been a theory that the cerebellum—known for motor coordination—might also be involved with emotional coordination.

Another objective and measurable result the study revealed was how the patient's nervous system reacted to listening to the description of their distressing event. The researchers used biofeedback equipment to measure the body's fight-or-flight response before and after NET treatments. The description of their event triggered a big fight-or-flight response before NET, but after NET their response was pretty much neutralized. This indicates that whenever there is a reminder of a distressing event, the fight-or-flight mechanism tends to get triggered. There is a substantial amount of research to corroborate that finding. Importantly, this chronic triggering then cascades into another set of physiological and psychological consequences, all leading to a less happy, less healthy life.

For example, as a part of Dr. Monti's study, the repetitive disruptions were measured with assessment tools such as traumatic stress scales, mood scales, anxiety scales, and quality-of-life scales. Many of the patients' scales registered way off the baselines. That's something to be expected, even though these patients had not said anything about psychological difficulties. What this tells us is that distressing events create a lot of traumatic stress regardless of whether it is noticeable to the patient. Burying it out of sight, out of mind doesn't work—just the opposite: trauma spreads its roots and grows into trees. In the language of the NET model, a distressing experience becomes a Neuro Emotional Complex (NEC), or to carry our metaphor further, an NEC grows into a patch of trees, or sometimes a forest. What surprised us about the results is how impactful even a brief NET intervention was on overall mood and psychological functions.

In looking back on your own life, what are the experiences you would prefer not to think about? Who wronged you so painfully that you get a sick feeling in your stomach when you think about them? What real or perceived failure do you not want anyone to know about because you still feel ashamed of it?

One key to resolving your NEC is to understand that it was not resolvable in that moment in time when it occurred—either there wasn't a solution then or the situation was too overwhelming for you, or both. Thus, your trauma got walled off. That's a good thing. Remember, survival is the driving force behind all this. Sometimes you consciously wall off—for instance: *I'll deal with it in the morning after I've slept on it.*

Other times it happens reflexively without your awareness—*Let's get out of this place. It's too crowded and too expensive*—when subconsciously you want to leave because you somehow associate it with your ex. That same NEC might cause you to subconsciously get a new job, jump into or out of a new relationship, change your worldview, and more, all under the guise of moving on, when really you're thrashing around trying to get unstuck from your ex.

There are endless ways an NEC can affect your decisions, behaviors, moods, accomplishments, and sense of well-being. Yet fixing it is not an easy task. Your brain doesn't like doing this, much the same way your body after a physical injury doesn't like the necessary exercises for rehabilitation. Also similar to a physical injury, an NEC often leaves scars.

You can try some NEC assessments on your own; below is the NET First Aid Stress Tool ("FAST") method for self-healing:

1. Identify an experience in your life that fits the description of an NEC—generally, that would be a distressing event.

2. Rate it on a scale from zero to ten, with zero being nonstressful and ten being the highest level of distress imaginable. Go through your various experiences until you find one that you rate as being greater than six.

3. Working with that greater-than-six NEC, identify the emotions you associate with it: fear, grief, sadness, anger, shame, disgust, interest, and joy. Since the last two are pleasurable emotions, usually they are not in play, so that narrows it down to six. Choose from those six—it's fine if there is only one. It is important to name the emotions and write them down.

4. Ask yourself, in the context of this upsetting event, what am I saying to myself about myself? Don't be surprised if your answers seem completely illogical. They usually will. They also will often be harsh judgments such as *I'm a bad person . . . it's me against the world,* and so on.

5. Go ahead and write it all down.

6. Once you have your emotions and self-referential statements in front of you, this allows the feeling and thinking parts of your brain to communicate with each other. Refer back to our NET study showing the parahippocampus area of the brain being highly charged before treatments. This area is where emotion-based memories are stored and where overactivation occurs when an NEC is triggered—the result is a relative disconnect from the reasoning centers in the neocortex, which means getting those two parts of the brain to communicate is half the battle.

7. Close your eyes and try to focus on your emotions and self-referential statements, then add in deep breathing, while placing one of your hands flat against your forehead and placing the first three fingers of the other hand on the pulse area of the hand that is on the forehead. In traditional Chinese medicine, this engages the major meridians (via the pulse points) and the emotional acupressure points in the forehead. Try to hold this focus as you take seven to ten deep breaths. Then switch hands so that you have the other one flat on the forehead while holding the pulse area of that wrist with the opposite hand, again for another seven to ten

breaths, staying as focused as possible on the emotions and self-referential statements. If you feel you need a few more breaths, that's fine too. You might notice an emotional release of some kind. This is usually the result of the present-day self now being part of the conversation and not completely disconnected from the emotional, illogical dialogue of the stressful event. You might also find that your brain went to other similar events in your life that carry the same theme, or you might have an "aha" moment. You might even notice some physical relaxation and hence a shift away from fight-or-flight. Any of these are healthful steps.

While this self-assessment doesn't incorporate all of the healing modalities of NET, it can be a helpful tool to combine with the other add-ons. Some of your distressing events, though, may be too stressful or too complex to address on your own. That's where a NET-certified practitioner utilizing the full intervention can make a big difference in your life.

Over the previous several years, the Marcus Institute has built a solid track record of success with the NET for treating patients who have suffered from traumatic or distressing events.[8]

Recommendation #3: Twelve-Step Program

We covered the basics of twelve-step programs in chapter 5; now we will get into the details of how it might help with resolving dysregulation resulting from toxic stress and trauma. While this aspect of twelve-step recovery is not its primary aim, it is the greatest healing that I received following decades of disordered eating. In the language of twelve-step, you could think of this quality as *emotional sobriety*.

In my forties, after nearly a decade as a member of a twelve-step fellowship,[9] what I found most compelling personally was that it introduced me to a daily spiritual program and provided the boundaries and accountability to follow through with it. Working the twelve steps provided a system for owning my part in my lack of emotional sobriety. Overall, twelve-step programs provide, as described in their literature, an operating manual for the inevitable ups and downs of life.

Natalie (not her real name to protect anonymity) explains, "Alcoholics Anonymous (AA) has provided me the tools for living life on life's terms. It isn't just about being sober, but being able to live with the knowledge and support needed to navigate the highs and lows of living. How to let things go, how to compartmentalize, how to pause and reflect and stay out of your head (it's a dangerous place!). AA is people just like you who aren't like you. All are welcome. All understand. All are experienced [and] have strength and hope. The AA fellowship is powerful, but YOU have to be willing, surrender, and work it because you are worth it."

Interestingly, one of the cofounders of Alcoholics Anonymous, Bill W, was a believer in the ability of LSD to provide spiritual breakthrough and recovery. As you might imagine, this is upsetting to some of the AA members, and details and sources are limited.[10]

I am grateful to be in recovery for fifteen years from disordered eating—restriction initially in high school (not quite meeting criteria for anorexia but certainly I was harming myself with caloric restriction), then bulimia in my twenties and thirties. Before you argue with me about whether food addiction exists, let me say that recovery has made all the difference in allowing me to eat in a way that is healthy and neutral. I finally eat the way that my body needs.

At age forty, I started a twelve-step program and immediately became "abstinent" with food. I lost twenty-five pounds and then discovered my lack of emotional abstinence, which in twelve-step we call "unmanageability." Even though my weight was normal at this stage, I still showed signs of dysregulated physiology, such as low heart rate variability and prediabetes—a state of high blood sugar, driven by my mind and perceived stress.

The structure of a food-based twelve-step program helped me stabilize my eating so that I was no longer restricting, bingeing, and purging. That led me to dive deeper into healing trauma and exploring addiction, recovery, and psychedelic medicine. It took me years to understand why I was so stuck with eating addictively, which is not the way that I wanted consciously to feed myself.

As I learned more about trauma and started to integrate what I discovered into my own life, to discuss it with my daughters, and then to bring it into patient care, I have come to agree with Stephen Porges, MD, the psychiatrist who developed polyvagal theory.[11] He contributed the idea that stress is not binary but that we have multiple states of stress, of nervous system activation (as we've covered in this book, I believe unresolved stress activates the entire PINE network, not just the nervous system). Polyvagal theory offers a fresh perspective on eating disorders that encompasses social connection in which eating reflects biological and behavioral state regulation. Dr. Porges adds that an eating disorder appears when ingestive behaviors replace social behavior as the main regulator of the autonomic state. Short version: some of us with trauma eat as a way to feel safe. It's a potentially effective strategy initially, but then it backfires if you're like me and you have physical, mental, emotional, and social consequences of disordered eating.

Dr. Porges's work rings true. There is part of me that learned to eat as a way to calm myself and feel safe. I would eat when I was stressed or happy or lonely. I had obsessive thoughts about food and food rituals, and spent hours each day planning my next meal, even healthy ones. I would eat to celebrate, poring over menus to find the perfect palate combinations. Food was recreation, love, entertainment. I would eat to change my emotional state. Carbs called to me the way that alcohol calls to others: bread, pasta, cookies, cake. Carbs raise serotonin and help you feel good in the moment, until you eat them addictively and they start to damage your metabolic health.

Now I don't use food in this way. I lean on daily tools to address trauma reactions, like yoga, meditation, prayer, mindfulness, Hakomi, being in nature, hydration, twelve-step tenets, and psychedelic-assisted therapy. What's difficult about food addiction is that you have to confront it several times per day with each meal, unlike other substances, like alcohol.

After gaining and losing about twenty-five to thirty pounds every few years from addictive patterns with food, including restricting and purging, I have now been at a stable weight for fifteen years. It feels like freedom. When I'm asked for the quick tip on how to resolve disordered eating, the truth is that there isn't one. You have to learn for yourself what the underlying drivers are and then address them. That's what makes eating disorders so difficult to treat.

Wrap-Up

We have witnessed an explosion of mind-body therapies over the past few decades, and I've only featured a few of the modalities with which I have had personal contact. There are many worth exploring that are not in this book, including various forms of meditation, hypnosis, guided imagery, yoga, Pilates, tai chi, Strozzi Institute, and countless others. As you learn to unpack the way that your body responds to stress, I encourage you to find the modalities that work best for you, and if you have a significant history of trauma and/or PTSD, find the modalities that are trauma-informed. Find the best trauma therapists in your area, and remember, some people need simultaneous medication since mind-body therapy can be a slow process.

CHAPTER 12

Everything You Want to Know About Psychedelics

Although many of us think of psychedelics as dangerous drugs, it's time for a rethink. They are non-toxic, non-addictive, have very few side effects, and could potentially offer relief for people suffering from a range of psychological difficulties.

—DR. ROSALIND WATTS, PHD, FOUNDER OF ACER INTEGRATION, CLINICAL PSYCHOLOGIST, AND CLINICAL LEAD FOR IMPERIAL COLLEGE PSILOCYBIN TRIAL

Justin, a young man suffering from long-standing depression, was born into an authoritarian Protestant household. Outwardly the family was successful in business and academics, with several sons being state champions in sports and attending top colleges. These hallmarks of success masked inward dysfunction and brutality. Punishments and degradation were the tools used to ensure conformity and to drive success in work, sports, and academics. The youngest of three boys, Justin faced beatings and neglect and witnessed spousal and alcohol abuse. His father created an age-based rank structure that incentivized the older brothers to beat their younger siblings without repercussions. At age five, Justin was stripped of all his clothes, toys, and belongings. He slept without clothing on a concrete floor in a closet under the stairs for weeks. To further ostracize him, Justin ate separately from the family, somehow subsisting on bread and cold leftovers. This crucible event forged a sense of extreme self-reliance but left him with PTSD and depression, while accelerating aging in his joints. As a young adult, he was diagnosed with osteoarthritis. His ACE score, using the Institute for Functional Medicine questionnaire, was seventeen, reflecting the serious abuse and neglect that he suffered as a child.

At age eighteen, Justin took a psychedelic called lysergic acid diethylamide (LSD, known colloquially as "acid"). Justin swallowed a so-called heroic dose (i.e., very high) of two LSD tabs and departed in a 1974 Jeep Wagoneer for a weekend mountain climbing and camping trip in a remote area of the Pacific Northwest wilderness. After arriving, Justin perceived the car swelling, breathing, and wrapping around him like a warm embrace as the LSD took effect (i.e., interacted with his hallucinogenic brain receptors, called serotonin-2A or $5\text{-HT}_{2A}\text{R}$), making him energized, euphoric, and full of awe while also distorting his visual perception. Hanging out in the car as the hours passed, Justin felt flickers of a new construct to his life. The predictions of failure and degradation from his family of origin came into a manageable focus. The LSD was providing what he sensed as a "top-down view" of his present life. For the first time he also was able to see new possibilities. He luxuriated in a newly found framework that showed him he could leave his town, family, and life behind. He felt an inward sense of contentment he'd never known.

Justin finally found the relief he most wanted on an acid trip. It was the reset that he needed to address the trauma that was unresolved inside of his body and save his life. While my advice in this chapter is to consider psychedelic-assisted treatment together with a trusted and experienced clinician to heal trauma, Justin did it on his own, recreationally with a friend. If you struggle with unresolved trauma that may be triggering chronic disease, whether that's autoimmunity or depression, heart disease or PTSD, psychedelic-assisted treatment is an important and novel solution to consider that has proven and durable effectiveness to help you provide resolution and re-create homeostasis in your system. In my opinion, after years of working in the field of psychedelic medicine with clients and patients, psychedelics offer the opportunity to address stuckness and restore resilience to the chronically stressed.

You will find that this chapter tends to emphasize the medical model of psychedelic treatment given the constraints currently placed on psychedelic use, and given my role as a medical doctor. You'll find that I am coloring carefully within the lines about a subject that does not color within the lines but asks you to start coloring outside of the lines with a state of awe and grace. I am aware of the irony and nuance.

As I will cover in this chapter, psychedelics are uniquely suited to help uncover and reprocess trauma, and sometimes unlearn the defensive patterns that worked at the time of the harm. I've personally witnessed this healing process time and again with ketamine, 3,4-methylenedioxy-methamphetamine (MDMA), and psilocybin. Not everyone has a first psychedelic experience like Justin's, but I commonly see what he experienced in my patients and clients as they:

1. See their own obstacles with greater clarity along with potential solutions;
2. Identify (and even abate) long-standing behaviors driven by trauma; and
3. Reframe their lives in a more rigorously honest way that no longer sacrifices authenticity for connection.

Increasingly, we are finding that nonordinary states of consciousness may reduce the harmful thought patterns in the brain that keep us hypervigilant and unhealthy and allow the entire system to confront difficult topics, reboot, form new memories, and potentially help with a host of ailments, from depression to autoimmunity.

What Are Psychedelics?

The word "psychedelic" means "soul, mind, or spirit manifesting," which one can think of as using thoughts, feelings, and beliefs to bring something into a current physical reality. Psychedelics are plant- and synthetic-based medications that trigger nonordinary (or, as some say, extraordinary) states of consciousness characterized by profound alterations in perception, emotion, spiritual availability, and cognition. The classic psychedelics include LSD, psilocybin ("magic mushrooms"), and mescaline. These are considered entheogens because people may experience awe; closeness to God, the divine, and/or Mother Nature; and dissolution of the separateness of oneself from other people. Another

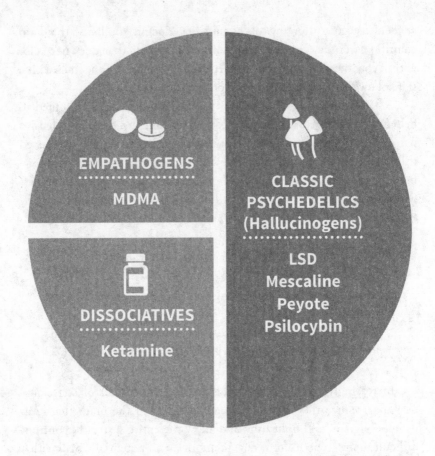

category of psychedelics is called empathogens because people feel more empathy (they can see others' points of view more easily, including gaining new perspective on their own experiences in childhood, as Justin experienced on LSD). One of the most well-studied empathogens, MDMA, has shown consistent evidence for helping people move past trauma. Another class of psychedelics is the dissociative medications of which ketamine is most well-known, showing great promise as a treatment for depression.

When we query people in the United States about their use of psychedelics, interesting patterns emerge. Overall, about 16 percent have tried psychedelics, with use rising as restrictions fall, especially for LSD and psilocybin.[1] Increased use has been associated with improved psychological functioning in both healthy volunteers and in patient populations, such as in people with PTSD and depression, likely due to increased neuroplasticity and improved cognitive flexibility.[2] Curiously, sometimes single doses, such as in Justin's case, can have beneficial effects lasting well past when they last used the medication (called durable effects).[3]

Meet the Most-Researched Psychedelics

After decades of misinformation and stigmatization, we are finally entering a new era of transparent and rigorous scientific inquiry on the benefits and safety of psychedelics and how they might offer better answers for those of us with trauma and its consequences, like autoimmunity. Here are the most proven psychedelics from a scientific perspective:

- **KETAMINE** was first synthesized in 1962 and regularly used as anesthesia, which is how I began working with it in the 1990s in the operating theater and emergency room. Ketamine is also used to treat depression, chronic pain, and suicide, and is being investigated for other indications, such as eating disorders and obsessive-compulsive disorder (OCD).[4] At low doses it acts as an empathogen, inducing feelings of relaxation, calm, and caring. At moderate doses, it can be hallucinogenic, and at higher doses it causes dissociation (you leave your body), which is how it's used in the operating theater, in the emergency room, and on the battlefield for wounded soldiers.
- **MDMA** (3,4-methylenedioxymethamphetamine, also known as Ecstasy or Molly) is a synthetic drug, invented in 1912 to help stop blood loss on the battlefield, and its use was restricted beginning in 1985. While not a classic psychedelic, MDMA acts figuratively as a heart-opening substance that facilitates social connection (hence the term "empathogen") with stimulant effects, producing an energizing quality, distortions in time and perception, and increased euphoria, empathy, emotional receptivity, compassion, and extroversion. Most importantly, MDMA reduces the activity of the limbic system in a manner that allows us to recall emotionally charged memories with much less emotional

intensity than historically is associated with revisiting these experiences. As a result, we are able to see different points of view and process the memory differently than in the past and in so doing have the potential to heal from these traumatic events. Studies have shown the medicine downregulates the limbic system (emotional center) and especially increases communication between the amygdala and hippocampus, enabling people to revisit previous traumatic experiences with less fear and emotional volatility. It is used primarily for patients with PTSD and OCD, in which the prosocial effects help reduce symptoms.[5] I find it very helpful for couples therapy too.

- **LSD** (lysergic acid diethylamide) is derived from a naturally occurring ergot alkaloid ergotamine and acts on serotonin, dopamine, and adrenaline pathways via receptors. It was vilified starting in the 1970s and fell victim to negative media that still prevails, and as a result, research has been severely limited. Most data are from small studies or uncontrolled recreational use. Overall, small studies of its potential therapeutic effects with addiction and depression have been positive, and it has been used for various reasons to help deepen therapy and to support trauma processing.[6] Dialing back in time to its initial heyday between the 1950s to 1970s, LSD was studied for the treatment of anxiety, depression, addiction, and pain in advanced cancer, in addition to augmentation of psychotherapy.[7] Before it went underground under the Nixon administration, even the esteemed *Journal of the American Medical Association* noted its clinical benefits.[8]

- **PSILOCYBIN**, also known as "magic mushrooms," is a chemical found in at least one hundred mushroom species and has been used by Indigenous cultures for centuries, particularly in Mexico and Central America.[9] For political reasons, most psychedelics, including psilocybin, were restricted to Schedule I in the early 1970s. According to the DEA, Schedule I is reserved for medications "with no currently accepted medical use and a high potential for abuse." Psilocybin is a classic psychedelic that, similar to LSD, activates serotonin receptors in the brain. Psilocybin is a potent antidepressant,[10] and it helps to reduce PTSD, alcohol use disorder, and potentially obsessive-compulsive disorder.[11] A recent study at Stanford of veterans with PTSD treated with psilocybin showed that 40 percent reported a significant positive effect.[12] Several described their trip as life-changing. A trial is underway for use in patients with fibromyalgia.[13] Similar to LSD, this substance has not been found to be addictive.

- **KANNA** is considered a sacred medicinal plant that acts as a natural mood booster, relieves stress, and promotes well-being. Some consider it a legal analog of MDMA, and though I am not yet convinced this is true from a scientific perspective, as I like to point out in all of my books, *lack of proof is not proof against.* Known by its scientific name, *Sceletium tortuosum*, kanna is indigenous to South Africa, specifically to the native San and Khoikhoi tribes. It was used historically by San hunter-gatherers and Khoi to reduce fatigue and for social, healing, and spiritual reasons.[14] Today, it is being tested for treatment of anxiety, depression, substance use disorders, and other psychological and psychiatric disorders.[15] Over the past fifteen years, various bioactive compounds have been isolated and classified from the plant, and science shows that the plant contains numerous anti-inflammatory, antimicrobial, antioxidant, antidepressant, neuroprotective, and anxiolytic effects.[16] Overall, the science is limited, including safety,[17] though thousands of years of use suggest a relatively safe track record.

- **CANNABIS** (What? Cannabis isn't a psychedelic, you say? Not so fast.) There is a growing movement—through ceremonial set and setting—to work with cannabis as a powerful health-promoting sacred plant medicine.[18]

How Do Psychedelics Work?

Many different lenses exist through which to see and understand how psychedelics work. For the purposes of this book, I will stay in the doctor's seat of Western science's current understanding, even as this may only complement or not reach other truths and ways of knowing, in particular traditional and Indigenous systems of knowledge, practice, and understanding.

From this place of Western science, we currently understand that psychedelics work via a network in the brain as I will detail below. In the Resources, I refer to other leaders, therapists, clinicians, and healers in this realm who offer a more expanded view.

Psychedelics work via specific brain pathways. Classic psychedelics act on the serotonin pathway, specifically via a receptor called serotonin 5-HT$_{2A}$ into which the psychedelic molecule fits like a key into a lock to induce many effects, including hallucinations, such as the visuals Justin experienced when the Jeep began hugging him. (Serotonin, or 5-hydroxytryptamine, is chemical that nerve cells produce, with complex functions that modulate mood, appetite, sleep, cognition, learning, memory, nausea and vomiting, and reward.)

The 5-HT$_{2A}$ receptor is found on the surface of many cells as well as inside the cell. It belongs to an entire family of serotonin receptors involved in learning, memory, and executive function in the brain, including nerve cells, or neurons, in the hippocampus (part of the brain involved in memory consolidation and emotional regulation), forebrain (cerebrum), and basal ganglia.[19] Sometimes problems with the structure and/or function of this serotonin receptor may be associated with conditions like anxiety, depression, addictive behaviors, attention deficit disorder, and schizophrenia.

While psychedelic-assisted treatment is now known to be highly effective at treating mental health problems related to trauma, it also helps healthy people enhance well-being and get unstuck. Why do psychedelics help healthy people? They increase neuroplasticity (or growth of new neural pathways) in parts of the brain that manage emotions, like the prefrontal cortex and hippocampus.[20]

In people with depression, psychedelics improve cognitive function. In addition to providing novel and nonordinary visual experiences, psychedelics reduce "rigid thinking" and sensitivity to the environment (allowing a person to be more present and less reactive or numb), and facilitate emotional release, especially emotions that have become stuck in the body. Ultimately, a person with depression may notice more creative thinking as they experience neuroplasticity.[21]

Preparation: Set, Setting, and Matrix

When preparing for a nonordinary state of consciousness with psychedelics, practitioners agree that set and setting are essential, as is the so-called matrix. Set and setting, at their simplest, refer to the mindsets of both the individual and their therapist/practitioner, with "set" including current state of mind, prior drug experiences that may influence their current state of mind, and their current mood. "Setting" refers to environmental factors in which the participant has their psychedelic session (i.e., the physical, social, and spiritual setting). "Matrix" refers to the "environment from which the subject comes: the environment surrounding the subject before and after the session, and the larger environment to which the subject returns."[22] Others have added "skill,"[23] and "support"[24] to the tasks of preparation.

Let me give you an example of set and setting from my own experience in a ceremony called a *velada*, which is a Mazatec healing vigil, usually led by a facilitator named a *curandera*, or traditional female folk healer. My mindset at the time was filled with anticipation and excitement, plus apprehension, because the ceremonial setting felt foreign to me. I had never been exposed to the cultural context from which she came, and this affected my experience during the session. I took part in the *velada* with eleven other people, mostly therapists, led by the *curandera*, who had traveled from Oaxaca, Mexico, to our remote location in Northern California. Our ceremony began at sunset. The *curandera* performed a ritual cleansing on each of us, gently brushing branches of rue (*ruda* in Spanish) and bay leaves against the fronts and backs of our bodies. Then I sat in a single bed with poofy pillows in a softly lit room, listening quietly as the *curandera* provided details about what to expect. Her assistant passed out a paper plate of mushrooms containing psilocybin to each of us. As we consumed the mushrooms with cacao beans and honey, as directed, the *curandera* recited the rosary so that the *Niños Santos* ("Holy Children," as mushrooms are known in Oaxaca by Mazatec healers, whose Indigenous traditions have intertwined with five hundred years of Christian colonialism) would reveal their spirit, alter our consciousness, and embed lasting healing and changes in our lives. While at first my initial set was anticipation, excitement, and apprehension, as I became familiar with our ceremony, I trusted the facilitator and relaxed into the experience.

Dose?

If psychedelics have the potential to improve brain neuroplasticity and reduce rigid thinking in people with depression, what dose is required to provide this effect? Do we need hallucinogenic doses, or do levels that don't dramatically change perception ("microdosing") help too?

- **MACRODOSING.** Justin took a hallucinogenic dose of LSD that was approximately 200 micrograms, which is what some but not all studies have found to increase growth factors in the brain such as brain-derived neurotrophic factor (BDNF).[25] Lower doses of LSD, in the range of 5 to 20 micrograms may likewise raise BDNF in the blood in healthy people.[26]

- **MICRODOSING.** While I do not recommend frequent large hallucinogenic doses of psychedelics because of their intensity and need for lengthy preparation, integration, and careful attention to set and setting, microdosing may be a different story. There are various protocols for microdosing, which can be done more frequently, such as every two to three days, and they are typically done to achieve a state change rather than trait change (state change results in a mood/attitudinal change in the moment with possibly short-term aftereffects, whereas a trait change results in persistent shift in mood/attitude enduring beyond the physiological effects of the medicine in the body).[27] Most people microdose as a way to self-manage their mental health.[28] The three most common microdosing medications are LSD, ketamine, and psilocybin. Some believe that nonhallucinogenic doses of psychedelics can enhance neuroplasticity, improve the PINE system, and augment personal growth, and research in the coming years may help evaluate the validity of this belief.[29]

What does the research show? One systematic review of forty-four studies of microdosing from 1955 to 2021 demonstrated improved pain perception, conscious state, and neurophysiology in some of the studies reviewed. One large study using psilocybin (n = 953) compared to non-microdosing controls (n = 180) showed improved mood.[30] Another large study of 6,753 people using low-dose psilocybin showed it was well tolerated, with a good safety record and a lack of side effects, and also showed benefits such as enhanced mood, creativity, focus, and sociability.[31]

Another small study of 278 subjects found microdosing improved mood and focus.[32] One randomized trial of 34 people showed that microdosing of psilocybin mushrooms results in mild subjective effects and altered brain waves (as measured by an electroencephalogram, or EEG), but there was not much evidence of enhanced well-being, creativity, or cognitive function.[33] Does microdosing psilocybin improve interoception (sensing, understanding, and feeling what's happening in the body)? Probably not.[34] In patients with depression, microdosing appears to be well tolerated, but it's not yet clear that it has a therapeutic benefit.[35] While the quality of the research is not great thus far, the few studies published have shown improved cognitive processing and mental health. These study outcomes used the research subject's self-report rather than relying on objective testing. At this time, it's premature to draw strong conclusions due to the bias, heterogeneity, and strong placebo effects, as well as inconsistencies in microdosing ranges across various substances.[36]

Further, the type of people who enroll in the current studies and those who choose to take a microdose seem to be different than people who are taking a hallucinogenic dose: they score lower on tests of dysfunctional attitude and negative emotionality, while scoring higher on tests of wisdom, open-mindedness, and creativity.[37]

In sum, there has been huge interest in microdosing with widespread participation in the United States. It has been a massive citizen scientist experiment with very few large-scale, well-designed trials to tell us the truth about how it works. We desperately need more rigorous research on microdosing with psychedelics with minimal bias and documentation of potential risks, if any.[38] We also need more studies to investigate whether chronic microdosing has different effects on neuroplasticity and rigid thinking compared to single, large doses. In particular, we need to know the potential risks of multiple administrations of psychedelics at the low-dose range, how they affect the PINE system, including physiology, mood, and mental health; how they impact cognitive function, such as memory and focus, creativity, personality, and consciousness; and if there are significant risks.

Risks

Certainly there are risks to taking psychedelics, though the potential harm is likely lower than one realizes,[39] and much less than those posed by alcohol.[40] Still, at the present moment, LSD, MDMA, and psilocybin are listed as Schedule I drugs by the federal government, which translates as "drugs with no currently accepted medical use and a high potential for abuse." Cannabis is still in this category as well, along with peyote. Classification of MDMA and psilocybin may change very soon if it hasn't already at the time of publication.

After years of criminalization, stigmatization, and the War on Drugs mantra, "Just say no," we are in a renaissance of renewed scientific and social interest in psychedelic medicine, and we are in a holding pattern as more data accumulate. Overall, most scientists agree that the risk of psychological distress and suicidality are reduced by psychedelic medicine when administered therapeutically.[41] One rigorous scientific review concluded, "Our review shows that medical risks are often minimal, and that many—albeit not all—of the persistent negative perceptions of psychological risks are unsupported by the currently available scientific evidence, with the majority of reported adverse effects not being observed in a regulated and/or medical context."[42] I agree. Be careful not to make decisions based on anecdotal evidence.

Still, I urge discernment. Some psychiatrists and experts believe that psychedelic-assisted therapy should be reserved for people who fail other conventional approaches.

If you have a psychiatric disorder managed by medication, such as selective serotonin reuptake inhibitors (SSRIs), consider evaluating the risks of drug interactions and serotonin toxicity associated with using both your prescribed medication and a psychedelic medication. Generally, serotonin toxicity is rare unless there is a drug overdose or a combination of two drugs that can increase intrasynaptic (inside the synapse or connection between nerve cells) serotonin and a drug that acts as a monoamine oxidase inhibitor (MAOI). Signs of serotonin toxicity warrant immediate medical attention and include rapidly changing vital signs, myoclonus (muscle jerks), shivering, agitation or comatose mental state, muscle rigidity, hyperthermia (fever), seizure activity, and in extreme cases, death.[43]

Here is a short list of the known risks of the medications, considered sacred by many, described in this chapter. My recommendation regarding risk is to discuss your personal risk with a trusted medical expert who is experienced with these medications and can advise you regarding personal safety.

- **KETAMINE** is used at higher doses as a dissociative anesthetic, but most people take it therapeutically at much lower doses, approximately 10 percent of the anesthetic dose. Depending on the dose administered, it is expected that you will experience distorted perception of sight and sound, potentially to the point of feeling disconnected from the body, detached from environment, and sometimes with loss of control. Additionally, at higher doses, you may experience an uncomfortable feeling of immobility (loss of motor control, including ability to talk), amnesia, high blood pressure, bladder irritation, and, rarely, laryngeal spasm (in less than 1 percent of patients). Keep in mind that ketamine is the anesthesia of choice for children in the emergency room for treating burns or mending broken bones, because it does not affect blood circulation or the respiratory system yet allows for dissociation between mind and body allowing doctors to treat the body without the patient experiencing discomfort or pain.
- **MDMA.** MDMA dramatically increases serotonin, dopamine, and oxytocin in the brain. Clinical studies suggest that MDMA puts some people at risk of high blood pressure, fainting, panic attacks, loss of consciousness, and seizures, which makes medical clearance prior to use essential, particularly for adults over the age of forty. When taken in a warm environment associated with vigorous physical activity, such as at a rave, there is risk of increasing body temperature, known as hyperthermia. Moderate doses of MDMA can interrupt the body's ability to regulate temperature, and that may lead to potentially life-threatening consequences such as electrolyte imbalances or brain swelling due to fluid retention, especially in women. Other more minor side effects are jaw clenching, restless legs, loss of appetite, depersonalization

(detachment from self), hot flashes, headache, sweating, and muscle or joint stiffness.

- **LSD.** As Justin experienced, large enough doses produce visual hallucinations and delusions, which, while for some may be a desired outcome, for others can be distressing and disorienting. Overdose may lead to psychosis, and while there is no known lethal dose of LSD, death can occur indirectly if the journeyer is not in a safe set and setting. Other adverse effects include nausea, loss of appetite, increased blood sugar, dry mouth, difficulty sleeping, tremors, and seizures.

- **PSILOCYBIN.** The effects of psilocybin may vary depending on species of mushroom, origin, growing and harvesting conditions, and how they are consumed. In general, psilocybin causes alterations of thought and perception, including of time, and thus among some consumers can cause panic and psychotic-like reactions at high dose. The most common side effect is psychological distress, which is why having a trusted psychedelic therapist is highly recommended for those inexperienced with this medicine. Other side effects include nausea and vomiting, drowsiness, impaired concentration, muscle weakness, poor coordination, unusual body sensations, paranoia, confusion, and scary hallucinations, although for some, these are considered part of the healing process. Some who take psilocybin may take a poisonous mushroom in error. Signs of mushroom poisoning include muscle spasms, confusion, and delirium—and any suggestion of this problem requires an immediate trip to the emergency room, as death can be an ultimate consequence. Some people experience headaches the next day. Set and setting are so important, and if not carefully attended, may cause a "bad trip."

Connecting the Dots: Psychedelics and Autoimmune Disease

We are at the beginning of a therapeutic relationship between psychedelics and autoimmunity treatment and prevention. I've seen it help people with autoimmune disease, such as Crohn's disease, rheumatoid arthritis, and long COVID, achieve remission. The future looks bright for psychedelic-assisted treatment because psychedelics are nonaddictive and have a well-demonstrated safety profile. We are moving toward a large body of work showing that in rigorous randomized trials, people are statistically and significantly better. While much is to be discovered, at the time of writing this book, I see three main therapeutic pathways for how psychedelics may influence people with autoimmune disease, and since MDMA is the closest to FDA approval, I've used it as the main example. Classic psychedelics will likely have similar effects based

PATHWAY	EVIDENCE
TRAUMA AND TOXIC STRESS RESOLUTION	• MDMA, in combination with therapy, may produce a window of tolerance that allows clients to revisit and process traumatic content without becoming overwhelmed by hyperarousal and dissociative symptoms.[44] • MDMA-assisted therapy may allow you to recall negative memories with more self-compassion.[45] • MDMA is prosocial and increases emotional engagement, which may enhance the therapeutic alliance, which may help treatment adherence and outcomes.[46]
INFLAMMATION MODULATION	• You can think of chronic inflammation as biochemical fear, and MDMA facilitates the processing and release of particularly intractable, potentially developmental, fear-related memories.[47] • MDMA can suppress innate immunity by lowering the activity of neutrophil (a type of white blood cell) and production of dendritic cell/macrophage-derived pro-inflammatory cytokines including tumor necrosis factor alpha, interleukin (IL)-1β, IL-12 and IL-15.[48]
NEUROPLASTICITY	• MDMA may reopen oxytocin-dependent neuroplasticity that typically closes after adolescence.[49]

THE FINE PRINT

You are probably wondering if any of these medicines are legal and whether you might need a trip to Amsterdam to experience psychedelic-assisted therapy. Fortunately, psychedelics may be part of the broader US medical system sooner than you think. Ketamine has been widely available for decades, though use is FDA approved as an anesthetic, and the nasal spray, called esketamine or S-ketamine, is approved for treatment-resistant depression.

The highest-quality evidence of randomized controlled trials supports the safety and effectiveness of MDMA for the treatment of PTSD and psilocybin for the treatment of depression, alcohol use disorder, cancer-related trauma, and anxiety. Other medicines for the treatment of psychiatric disorders, such as using LSD and ayahuasca in a therapeutic setting, is in the early stages, though it's promising.

We suspect that MDMA will be FDA approved in mid-2024, making it available by prescription nationwide. Psilocybin is next in line. Meanwhile, at the state level, legal issues vary widely. In 2020, Oregon voters approved Measure 109, the Oregon Psilocybin Services Act, the first law in the United States that provides a regulatory system for receiving psilocybin, and psilocybin service centers in Oregon began opening their doors in 2023. Further, in Colorado, it is legal for people twenty-one and older to possess, share, and use psilocybin.

MDMA is illegal and, as described earlier, a Schedule I substance under the Controlled Substances Act. LSD is also Schedule I. (Again, Schedule I drugs are considered to have high abuse potential and no legitimate medical purpose though neither has been demonstrated in psychedelic-assisted therapy trials.)

Ketamine-assisted therapy is widely available, and a quick google search will help you find a worthy prescriber and therapist in your area. Sometimes you'll find both prescriber and therapist in a single person, like a psychiatrist who has performed advanced training in ketamine and also provides therapy, but most of the time, you'll see two different clinicians.

Importantly, in the context of psychedelic-assisted therapy, these are not the typical psychiatric medicines that are taken daily. Instead, as in the case of MDMA, the treatment consists of two to three sessions with MDMA with preparation sessions and integration sessions before and after. This represents a new paradigm in treating psychiatric illness and, as I've emphasized, may help alleviate physical symptoms too.

on their interaction with serotonin receptors, since serotonin is a brain chemical that is involved in psychological states, such as happiness, satisfaction, and optimism, and physiological states, such as appetite, sexual desire, and sleep.[50] Additionally, psychedelic medicines affect the way systems of the brain work together, creating more connections in parts of the brain that don't routinely communicate and an overall healthier groove—which many perceive as a healing state of consciousness.[51]

Wrap-Up

In my opinion from coaching dozens of people using psychedelic medicine as a therapeutic tool, the altered state of consciousness achieved provides a unique healing opportunity. Concierge and integrative physician Bradly Jacobs, MD, has described this concept as "healing states of consciousness."[52] I have witnessed people gaining the capacity to confront difficult life circumstances with more ease than typically experienced. Self-doubt, rumination, and maintaining a more limited view of oneself is replaced with more assuredness, confidence, clarity of intention, and grasping of a larger perspective surrounding their circumstances.

As a result, they are more at ease and experience steady progress that is durable. When you combine these—what many consider to be sacred—medicines with safe and effective integration therapy, you feel safer, your pain and your "story" of what's in your way soften, and you can create a new, healthier relationship to your past. We have much more to learn about how they work and when they can help, but if you suffer from autoimmunity and trauma, consider talking to your primary care doctor, health-care team, and/or therapist about what might be right for you.

Risk is low, and despite aggressive drug laws with heavy penalties, policy is finally changing. As a result, you may be wondering about the logistics of how to access the healing states of consciousness that may be achieved with these medicines. My advice is to start with your primary care provider and to track the progress of MDMA and psilocybin as they traverse the FDA landscape and become more widely available. Keep the vision broad and deep, and consider too the mystical and metaphysical qualities of sacred medicines and how you might want to consider developing a relationship with them.

CHAPTER 13

Your Autoimmune Blueprint

*It's in bringing others the healing gifts we've received that
the benefits of these gifts become truly ours.*

—ALBERTO VILLOLDO, PSYCHOLOGIST,
MEDICAL ANTHROPOLOGIST, AND SHAMAN

Jane is a forty-seven-year-old entrepreneur, wife, and mother of two teenagers experiencing perimenopausal symptoms superimposed upon a long history of premenstrual dysphoric disorder (PMDD). She has several serious cardiometabolic health concerns on laboratory testing related to cholesterol and blood sugar plus an elevated coronary artery calcium score. When combined with a strong trauma history, as we've explored, the cardiometabolic problems and toxic stress are probably related. Jane and I have been acquainted for eighteen years and met initially in a prenatal yoga class when we were pregnant with our daughters who are now heading to college. Her adverse childhood experience (ACE) score is nine, theoretically putting her at grave risk of stiffening of the arteries, cardiovascular disease, and premature death, among other problems.[1] Usually women do not develop heart disease until after menopause—did Jane have it established already, at such a young age?

For Jane, trauma probably drove her academically and professionally toward achievement, productivity, and at times hyperindependence, a trauma state described as *superautonomous self-sufficiency*. Trauma has varied effects. Not all who experience an elevated ACE score develop these high-performing traits. Many people subjected to trauma lose their full capacity, contributing to overwhelm, a fawn ("please and appease") response, and potentially underperformance. What is true for you? Are you hyperindependent, taking on too much and declining help, noticing that you have trouble with delegating to others?

Like Jane, I certainly used to struggle with these traits myself. Hyperindependent traits are often a downstream consequence of trauma, develop without your conscious awareness, and may combine with hypervigilance in a way that sets one up for dysregulated physiology and a greater risk of chronic disease, including the number one killer of men and women: coronary artery disease. Hyperindependent traits are highly valued in dysfunctional families and relationships because it makes a child, adolescent, and adult much easier to manage when they have few to no needs, and these traits continue to be highly valued in educational and work systems.

As a result, the trauma response, be it hyperindependence or addiction, or overwhelm, or even not living in alignment with your actual capacity, passion, and purpose, gets reinforced until a person decides consciously to interrupt the pattern. The problem, of course, is that when the trait and associated behaviors are a consequence of trauma, many of us don't trust well, self-sabotage, and suppress our true emotions in relationships, with compromised attachment to others.

Despite her young age, Jane has cholesterol problems (now presumed to be associated with trauma[2]), blood sugar dysfunction (as we've covered, a common finding in people with significant trauma[3]), and an elevated coronary artery calcium score, an indicator of established heart disease and calcified plaque in the coronary arteries of her heart. Trauma is a social determinant of health and inflammation,[4] particularly in people with a greater genetic risk of cardiometabolic disease.[5] Her low-density lipoprotein and apolipoprotein B are high, reflective of greater risk of cardiovascular disease, while her high-density lipoprotein, thought to be protective, is low. Uric acid, an important indicator of metabolism, is high. The stress hormone cortisol is high.

Some experts consider Jane's cardiovascular disease to be a form of autoimmunity, particularly microvascular disease of the coronary arteries in which the body attacks the lining of the blood vessels.[6] While the development of coronary artery disease is complex, the emerging view of it is that it is a type of vascular autoimmune condition. That means the immune system is attacking the blood vessel wall. Additionally, most autoimmune disease is an atypical risk factor for cardiovascular disease, so the risk is bidirectional.[7]

As an athlete and Bay Area foodie who ate a nutritious diet, Jane was shocked. Her father died prematurely of heart disease at age forty-two, so she sought early care to make sure she wouldn't meet the same fate.

Jane explains, "When I first discovered that I had a calcium score that placed me in the ninetieth percentile for my age and gender for risk of a heart attack, along with elevated cholesterol, I was alarmed and confused. I was a healthy, active woman who paid attention to my nutrition, and I had completed an Ironman-distance triathlon just years before. I first assumed that it was all genetics since my father had died at forty-two, not surviving his third heart bypass operation. This test result came just a few months before I started experiencing perimenopause and the associated hormonal disruptions, which were accompanied by raging anxiety attacks, nightmares, and more (which I've since realized were PTSD symptoms). As I started to seek help for these multiple issues, a few different pathways emerged that led me to understand that while genetics played a role in my health outcomes, it wasn't nearly the whole story."

Jane kicked her lifestyle management into high gear to address her cholesterol issues, heart disease, and blood sugar. She started wearing a continuous glucose monitor to guide the way she eats, with a renewed daily focus on organic food and colorful, fiber-rich vegetables that stabilize her blood sugar. She removed sugar and gluten, and other foods that spike her glucose. She's in bed by ten p.m. and follows strict sleep hygiene strategies. She uses eco- and body-friendly cosmetics and cleaning products in her home. She's reduced stress dramatically. Fitness has become more targeted—Ironman triathlons have been replaced with exercise that downregulates her nervous system, such as daily yoga, zone two training, power cardio, lots of walking, and preservation and building of muscle mass—and fortunately, these types of exercise have been shown to help both one's psychology and related physiology in women with adverse childhood experiences. And she worked with psychedelic medicines.

Importantly, she made several trauma-related discoveries while receiving MDMA-assisted therapy. In her words, "Doing MDMA-assisted therapy exposed years of childhood trauma and abuse that I'd only peripherally allowed myself to think about over the course of my forty-seven years. The sessions led to discoveries of physical, sexual, and emotional abuse at the hands of my mother and brother. With careful integration and a lot of support, I have been able to heal these wounds and start to rebuild a life defined by all-new metrics of ease and well-being, as opposed to one defined by productivity and relentlessly proving my worth. This process also exposed me to the relationship of adverse childhood experiences to physical disease which I hadn't previously been aware of and which I now believe were active contributors to my calcium score, cholesterol, decades of PMDD, and more. Exploring the spiritual dimensions of life through meditation and other insight practices has yielded an internal peace I could only have dreamed of and had no idea was attainable. The combination of MDMA and ketamine therapy, psychotherapy, psychopharmacology, and Western medicine has brought me to a place of sheer enthusiasm for life and a seemingly boundless vitality."

Jane has experienced great healing as she implements advanced therapies to address her health trajectory. Her cholesterol is substantially improved. Her blood sugar is now in the normal range. Our hope is to reverse her coronary artery calcium score, a possibility that has been documented in some individuals. However, it hasn't all been a steady march to reclaiming health. After one of her MDMA-assisted therapy sessions, she found that the mind-body therapies of brainspotting and EMDR, described in chapter 5, caused an uncomfortable destabilization of her brain networks, which is a potential risk of the pattern disruption of trauma work. This is one of the risks of any type of therapy. Her response occurs sometimes in people who are recovering from trauma. Jane was able to slow down and halt therapy for a while to find her own pace and regain a sense of calm and containment, but the process was frightening. Jane and I hope that sharing her full experience will serve as tempered encouragement for others, and noting that in trauma recovery, it's best not to do too much too soon. Find the right pace for you.

In this final chapter, I want to invite you to accept the opportunity presented to you in this book—to measure your trauma, consider not only mental health but also physical health aspects of your trauma level, and start to identify the subtle and not-so-subtle ways that an unresolved stress response may be dysregulating your psycho-immuno-neuro-endocrine (PINE) system. Once you understand your stress response, you can pick from the protocols in this book to begin the challenging inner work that is at the heart of trauma recovery. Advanced therapies like psychedelics give us an incredible opportunity to repattern the network of the body, but you have to meet them in the middle, that is, do your work. My aim is to reassure you that you are capable, to help you find trusted allies and partners on this journey, and to encourage you to take the first step.

Putting Together Your Blueprint for Healing: Who, What, Where, When, How?

You might have a lot of questions about how to implement the therapies in previous chapters, such as how to find the best Hakomi therapist, what immunomodulators to try, or even whether you really need to eliminate dairy in order to quell the unresolved immune response of autoimmunity. I get it. This chapter is designed to guide you through the final bits so that you can customize the autoimmune blueprint for you and create healing.

Regarding where to start, most people begin with the elimination diet and follow it for three weeks to three months, depending on the severity of their symptoms. Then they layer on top the suggestions from the sleep and toxic stress chapter. If you have autoimmune disease or pre-disease, you might then add on immunomodulators, or mind-body therapies. Alternatively, you could pick the area that is most problematic for you, such as food or toxic stress. Start there with the suggestions in that chapter for a week or two to get your bearings, then layer on another protocol.

I do not recommend jumping first to psychedelic medicines—you'll get the greatest benefit if you first establish a therapeutic foundation by preparing your body and understanding the issues related to trauma-induced dysregulation.

You've learned in the pages of this book how trauma can rewire your body to trigger autoimmune diseases—and we have covered a comprehensive plan for you to reset your psycho-immuno-neuro-endocrine (PINE) system and finally heal.

The important thing is not to wait until the perfect moment, but to just jump in and start. In previous books, I've written about the idea that imperfect action trumps perfect inaction, paraphrased from other wise souls. Given that trauma drives us to wait until the perfect moment, my wish for you is to dive in and get started even if the process is imperfect.

When I was in twelve-step, I learned that the most important question for spiritual development is "How?," not "When do I start the elimination diet?" (though it is important to commit to a date). Instead of asking, "Who is my therapist?" ask yourself, "How do I surrender to this process and create the type of healing that I most want for myself?" and "What is my vision for my future self, fully healed?" Those are the questions that can pull you forward to wholeness.

We Heal Individually and Communally

We know that social connection is essential to health, and trauma makes this especially true. There was a study sponsored by Cigna that showed social connection is essential to health, yet loneliness is at an all-time high.[8] The researchers found that only half of Americans in 2019 were having meaningful daily face-to-face interactions, and I imagine it's only declined from there since the pandemic.

If we take the lowering of mortality as a proxy for an important outcome, studies show that exercise lowers mortality by 20 percent and good diet by 30 percent, but relationships and having friends and being connected to community can lower mortality by 45 percent.

Maybe it's the fact that I'm now in my fifties, but increasingly I feel a new opportunity to wake up from the trance that we are separate and that materialism is our primary goal. COVID-19 encouraged many of us to enter a time of deep exploration of restorative justice, with respect to racism, imperialism, and colonialism.

While this book is primarily about an individual's response to trauma—how it can dysregulate the psycho-immuno-neuro-endocrine network, leading to autoimmune disease, allergic responses, and persistent symptoms—it is also about how what happens to the individual happens to the collective.

Collective trauma refers to the consequences of a shared traumatic event or systemic oppression of a group, like a culture or community. Examples include slavery and the genocide of Native Americans in the United States, the Nanjing Massacre, the Holocaust, the Armenian genocide, Pearl Harbor, the atomic bombings of Hiroshima and Nagasaki, the September 11, 2001, terrorist attacks, and even the COVID-19 pandemic. Collective trauma changes history and becomes embedded in the psychology and biology—the mind and body—of many who experience it. Sequelae of collective trauma mirrors individual trauma with increased panic, anxiety, depression, grief, toxic stress, and post-traumatic stress disorder visible at the population level.

As a corollary, the individual is part of the collective, and so an individual's trauma aggregates to contribute to collective trauma. Fortunately, the conduit connecting the individual and the collective is not only for transmission of trauma, but also for healing from it. As we learn how to regulate the body with healing practices, we can become beacons of regulation for others. This "coregulation" is the ability of your individual actions to modify the experience of another person. A classic example is how an infant is calmed by a parent's regulation, which is shared through, for example, skin-to-skin and heart-to-heart contact. Coregulation is not confined to infancy or childhood. I use coregulation with my patients or when my daughter is upset and needs support—I offer a warm relationship, a soothing environment, and I slow down my breathing. All this takes place before I offer skills instruction and coaching, because these secondary offerings need to arise through relationship—how can I know what to offer or have my offering received if we are not tuned to each other?

Lilla Watson, a Murri (Indigenous Australian) activist, artist, and academic working in Aboriginal epistemology, captured the need for coregulation to heal collective trauma: "If you have come here to help me, you are wasting your time, but if you have come because your liberation is bound up with mine, then let us work together."

While we each need to do our part to heal ourselves, we can also draw upon collective tools such as coregulation to heal not only ourselves but also our collective trauma. Coregulation begins with body care and awareness so that we have the capacity for the attunement. Just like a plant that needs safety, support, and the right conditions to flourish, our bodies need these things too. Importantly, we can hold more together than we can individually.

Behavior Change

While we've come far in our understanding of the underpinnings of autoimmunity and what might help to reverse disease, the most important work is to follow through and actually do the things. Behavior change is key to your success with implementing the autoimmune blueprint and healing your autoimmune condition. As Jane did, you must take personal responsibility for your health in order to get well.

Making behavior change stick is a fascinating topic. While a full discussion is beyond the reach of this book, I encourage you to understand briefly the what, the how, and the techniques for making it stick, as I've learned to do from a concierge medicine colleague, Bradly Jacobs, MD,[9] which draws upon the work of BJ Fogg,[10] a professor and behavioral scientist at Stanford University.

- **WHAT:** What is one thing you want to start doing or do more of (e.g., measure your ACE score, perform an elimination diet, start practicing Holotropic Breathwork®, begin Hakomi therapy, sleep better, find a prescriber for low-dose naltrexone or perhaps ketamine-assisted therapy)? What is the ultimate goal? What is the reward? What is the specific behavior to which you are committing?
- **HOW:** How will you cue the new behavior (example: set an alarm at nine thirty p.m. that it's time to get ready for an early bedtime)? How could you get thrown off from your new behavior? How will you adjust when something throws you off?
- **MAKING IT STICK:** What will help keep you motivated along the way? What are small milestones that you can accomplish without feeling overwhelmed? Who or what can help you remain accountable?

Complete each of these steps by answering the questions and finding an ally who can help you stay accountable. As Jane's story showed, one needs to take personal responsibility in order to get well. True, but what underlies not taking personal responsibility in the first place? There's a tautology that would be helpful to break out of; by definition, traumatized people often don't take care of themselves in some way. This may be one of the most important roles of healing states of consciousness: to get people popped out of the tyranny of trauma so that they can claim their life—their right to thrive.

Wrap-Up

We started this book by connecting the dots between autoimmunity and trauma, and we've broadened the definition of "trauma" and the unresolved stress response that it creates in the body. In my twenty-five years of practicing medicine, I was humbled to learn that my skills were insufficient to address the needs of my clients and patients. I discovered how dysregulated my own system was in the face of conflict and re-creations of the trauma of my childhood, which got me curious about the neurobiological effects of conflict in my clients and patients. In the past few years, I've optimized my microbiome with foods and supplements, and I mostly abstain from alcohol. I also have dedicated myself to the deep and challenging opportunity of opening my aperture to live beyond trauma and into growth that is provided by reverent practice with psychedelic medicines such as low-dose naltrexone, ketamine, and MDMA, and sacred plants, including psilocybin mushrooms.

Now I feel more, I tolerate less bad behavior from others, and I'm much more clear on how I want to live my life. My autoantibodies are gone, at least the nonspecific ones that I track, like antinuclear antibodies. I am now certified in psychedelic-assisted medicine with MDMA, psilocybin, and ketamine, but not everyone needs psychedelics to achieve healing states of consciousness.

My advice is to ask yourself if you have trauma that you need to address, which may be showing up in your body, symptoms, laboratory tests, and/or relationships. Let the wisdom of your body's sensations allow you to access and release the trauma that is held in your tissues. Pick a protocol that speaks to you in terms of bottom-up healing. The reason there are so many protocols to choose from in this book is that you not only need to find the right pace, you also need to find the right fit. Not all of the protocols in this book will be equally effective for you. That's why I want for you to work with a trusted, collaborative, and experienced clinician or practitioner who can guide and help tailor the best treatments to your particular context and perhaps physiology.

ACKNOWLEDGMENTS

My greatest thanks go to my patients, clients, and cases in this book. Together we are redefining the role of trauma in dysregulation and loss of health, so that we can reclaim wellness and healing for ourselves and others. Thank you for teaching me more about trauma and the intersection of mental and physical health, and for collaborating with me in such fulfilling work.

Books are a labor of love and vision. Thank you to Deb Brody, vice president and editorial director at Harvest, part of the HarperCollins Publishers/William Morrow Group. It's our second book together with my wise and talented editor, Sarah Pelz. Endless gratitude to Liate Stehlik, president and publisher of William Morrow Group at HarperCollins, for making this book possible.

I am grateful to my literary team, including my brilliant agent, Celeste Fine; my gifted editor, John Maas; and many others on the Park Fine Literary and Media team, including Sarah Passick and Mia Vitale. Thank you to my internal team of Nathali Hadi, Sharon Kastoriano, and Kenny Gregg.

This book would not be possible without the enduring support of many important people: Doug and Rachel Abrams, the staff and board at the Academy of Integrative Health & Medicine, Elena Brower, Anu French, Cynthia Good, Glendon Good, David Gottfried, Maya Gottfried, Allison Hagey, Victoria Hall, Johanna Ilfeld, Bradly Jacobs, Sandy Kleiman, Jeff Krasno, Heather Kuiper, Jenny Cundari, Keith Kurlander, Renske Lynde, Casey Means, Natalie Monetta, Daniel Monti, Leslie Murphy, Tamara Neuhaus, Andy Newberg, Mark Nicolson, Gemma Null, Davi Pakter, Meagan Pi, Justina Phillips, Laura Pontiggia, Nathan Price, Anna Reed, Zach Shimon, Maria Shriver, Larry Smarr,

Cary Sparks, Albert Szal, Mary Szal, Elizabeth Thomas, William Van Derveer, Pam Walter, Jenni Wendell, Martin Wood, Laura Woodrow.

Thank you to the scientists, therapists, practitioners, and psychonauts who have paved the way for the renaissance of psychedelic medicine and other ways to access healing states of consciousness.

Last, I am in awe of the potential of sacred plants to help us all evolve toward greater understanding, coregulation, interdependence, and relationship. Ultimately, when revered and used accordingly in ceremony, they are the true healers in transformative work.

GLOSSARY

ADVERSE CHILDHOOD EXPERIENCES (ACEs)—trauma that occurs during childhood, including emotional, physical, or sexual abuse and household dysfunction during childhood

ANTINUCLEAR ANTIBODIES (ANAs)—antibodies against the nucleus of cells

AUTOANTIBODIES—antibodies made by immune cells against substances or tissues formed by the person's own body

AUTOIMMUNITY—a condition in which the immune system is attacking normal tissues in the body, classically associated with autoantibodies against the tissue

CEREBELLUM—the region of the brain in the back of the head between cerebrum and brain stem, thought to control solely complex motor functions like walking but more recently found to be involved in trauma

CROHN'S DISEASE—an autoimmune condition that's a type of inflammatory bowel disease and causes chronic inflammation, scarring, and strictures of the gastrointestinal tract

EHLERS-DANLOS SYNDROME—a group of inherited disorders that affect your connective tissues, primarily skin, joints, and blood vessels

FIBROMYALGIA—a chronic condition that involves widespread muscle pain and discomfort, accompanied by fatigue, sleep disruptions, and poor memory and mood

HAKOMI—a form of mindfulness-based somatic therapy, also described as assisted self-study

HASHIMOTO'S THYROIDITIS—an autoimmune disorder affecting the thyroid gland and the most common cause of hypothyroidism, or low thyroid function

HIPPOCAMPUS—an important and complex brain structure embedded in the temporal lobe; plays a critical role in learning, emotional regulation, and memory

INCREASED INTESTINAL PERMEABILITY—also known as leaky gut; refers to the lining of the intestines, designed to absorb nutrients and water from food and place them in the bloodstream; but some people have excess permeability so that the lining leaks. One of the triad in the root cause leaky gut along with genetic susceptibility and trigger(s).

INTEROCEPTION—one's capacity to sense internal signals from your body, such as when you are thirsty or your heart is beating fast

KETAMINE—also known as K or Special K; a psychedelic and dissociative medication regularly used as anesthesia, now used at lower doses to treat depression, chronic pain, and suicide, among other conditions

LSD—lysergic acid diethylamide, also known as acid; classic psychedelic medicine that acts on serotonin, dopamine, and adrenaline pathways via receptors

MDMA—3,4-methylenedioxymethamphetamine, also known as Ecstasy or Molly; a synthetic drug whose use was restricted beginning in 1985. While not a classic psychedelic, MDMA acts figuratively as a heart-opening substance that facilitates social connection (hence the term "empathogen") with stimulant effects, producing an energizing quality, distortions in time and perception, and increased euphoria, empathy, emotional receptivity, compassion, and extroversion.

N-OF-1—an experiment whereby a person serves as their own control, with *n* being the study's sample size—in this case, one person

NEURO EMOTIONAL TECHNIQUE (NET)—a holistic mind-body approach for exploring and releasing stress-related conditions in the body

POST-TRAUMATIC STRESS DISORDER (PTSD)—a condition in which an individual has trouble recovering from a traumatic exposure

PRECISION MEDICINE—medical care that targets optimal benefit for a particular patient or group of patients by using genetic, molecular, and biomarker profiling

PSILOCYBIN—(also known as magic mushrooms) a psychedelic found in at least one hundred mushroom species that has been used by Indigenous cultures for centuries, particularly in Mexico and Central America

PSORIASIS—an autoimmune condition in which skin cells accumulate and form itchy, dry patches

PSYCHEDELIC(S)—"psychedelic" means "soul, mind, or spirit manifesting," which one can think of as using thoughts, feelings, and beliefs to bring something into a current physical reality. Psychedelics are plant- and synthetic-based medications that trigger nonordinary states of consciousness characterized by profound alterations in perception, emotion, spiritual availability, and cognition.

RHEUMATOID ARTHRITIS (RA)—an autoimmune chronic inflammatory disorder that affects several joints. People with rheumatoid arthritis suffer with painful swelling of the joints, erosion of the bone, and changes in the shape (sometimes deformity) of the joint.

SJÖGREN'S SYNDROME—an autoimmune disease characterized by dry eyes and dry mouth

TRAUMA—an unresolved stress response, sometimes a chronic freeze or immobilized state, that constricts the capacity of a person to respond in the present moment from the authentic self.

TWELVE-STEP PROGRAM—a program supporting recovery from substance use disorder, behavioral addiction, and compulsions, developed originally in the 1930s as Alcoholics Anonymous

TYPE 1 DIABETES (T1D)—an autoimmune condition in which the pancreas produces little or no insulin owing to autoimmune attack of islet cells

ULCERATIVE COLITIS (UC)—an autoimmune condition that is a type of inflammatory bowel disease that causes inflammation in the innermost lining of the large intestine (colon) and rectum.

NOTES

Introduction

1. Radha had the following abnormalities on her blood test:
   Total cholesterol 279 mg/dL (optimal < 200)
   High triglycerides (TG), a type of fat, at a level of 144 mg/dL (optimal < 100)
   High low-density lipoprotein or LDL 195 mg/dL (optimal < 100)
   Borderline low high-density lipoprotein, or HDL 54, which makes me want to check HDL function (optimal > 50)
   TG/HDL 2.7 (optimal <2)
   LDL Particle (LDL P) 2633 nmol/L (optimal <900)
   ALT 31 U/L (optimal <20)
   Vitamin D, 25-Hydroxy 25.7 ng/mL (optimal 60–90)
   Fasting glucose 104 mg/dL (from 2015, optimal < 85)
   Fasting insulin 14.1 mU/L
   TSH 4.48 uIU/mL (from 2015, optimal 0.3–2.5)
   High-sensitivity C-reactive protein 3.9 mg/L
   Homocysteine 9.2 umol/L
   Oxidative LDL 60 U/L
   Neutrophil-to-lymphocyte ratio as high as 6.4 in the past (2015)
   For my patients and clients, I recommend high-sensitivity C-reactive protein of < 1.0 mg/L, homocysteine of 5 to 7 umol/L, oxidative LDL (oxLDL) < 60, and neutrophil-to-lymphocyte ratio < 1.0.
2. I. Gardoki-Souto et al., "Prevalence and Characterization of Psychological Trauma in Patients with Fibromyalgia: A Cross-Sectional Study," *Pain Research and Management* (2022).
3. I am a clinical assistant professor in the Department of Integrative Medicine & Nutritional Sciences at Thomas Jefferson University. To learn more, go to https://www.jeffersonhealth.org/conditions-and-treatments/executive-health and/or https://www.jeffersonhealth.org/find-a-doctor/g/gottfried-sara.
4. SR Dube et al., "Cumulative Childhood Stress and Autoimmune Diseases in Adults," *Psychosomatic Medicine* 71, no. 2 (2009): 243.

5. M. Dong et al., "Insights into Causal Pathways for Ischemic Heart Disease: Adverse Childhood Experiences Study," *Circulation* 110, no. 13 (2004):1761–66.

6. M. Rizzo, RT Rossi, O. Bonaffini, C. Scisca, G. Altavilla, L. Calbo et al., "Increased Annual Frequency of Hashimoto's Thyroiditis Between Years 1988 and 2007 at a Cytological Unit of Sicily," *Annales d'Endocrinologie* 71, no. 6 (2010): 525–34, doi:10.1016/j. ando.2010.06.006.
   J. Xu, K. Ding, L. Mu et al., "Hashimoto's Thyroiditis: A 'Double-Edged Sword' in Thyroid Carcinoma," *Frontiers in Endocrinology* 13 (February 24, 2022): 801925, doi:10.3389/fendo.2022.801925.

7. SY Lee and EN Pearce, "Assessment and Treatment of Thyroid Disorders in Pregnancy and the Postpartum Period," *Nature Reviews Endocrinology* 18, no. 3 (2022): 158–171, doi:10.1038/s41574-021-00604-z.

8. S. McDonald et al., "N-of-1 Trials in Healthcare," *Healthcare* 9, no. 3 (2021): 330.

9. B. Brown, "TED Talk: The Power of Vulnerability" (2010), October 2, 2023, https://www.ted.com/talks/brene_brown_the_power_of_ vulnerability?utm_campaign=tedspread&utm_medium=referral&utm_ source=tedcomshare.

10. Known as the ecological fallacy. P. Sedgwick, "Understanding the Ecological Fallacy," *BMJ* 351 (2015): h4773.

11. Known as the atomistic fallacy. AV Diez Roux, "A Glossary for Multilevel Analysis," https://jech.bmj.com/content/56/8/588.

Chapter 1: The Autoimmunity Epidemic

1. National Institutes of Health, The Autoimmune Diseases Coordinating Committee, "Progress in Autoimmune Diseases Research," https://www .niaid.nih.gov/sites/default/files/adccfinal.pdf.

2. In autoimmune disease, the underlying problem is that the immune system has lost its ability to distinguish self antigens from non-self antigens. Note that antigens are a molecule or foreign matter, like a splinter, that can bind to an antibody or an immune cell.

3. AE Gracia-Ramos et al., "New Onset of Autoimmune Diseases Following COVID-19 Diagnosis," *Cells* 10, no. 12 (2021): 3592; M. Al-Beltagi et al., "COVID-19 Disease and Autoimmune Disorders: A Mutual Pathway," *World Journal of Methodology* 12, no. 4 (2022): 200; JM Anaya et al., "Is Post-COVID Syndrome an Autoimmune Disease?," *Expert Review of Clinical Immunology* 18, no. 7 (2022): 653–66; M. C. Sacchi et al., "SARS-CoV-2 Infection as a Trigger of Autoimmune Response," *Clinical and Translational Science* 14, no. 3 (2021): 898–907; M. Rojas et al., "Autoimmunity Is a Hallmark of

Post-COVID Syndrome," *Journal of Translational Medicine* 20, no. 1 (2022): 1–5; Y. Acosta-Ampudia et al., "Persistent Autoimmune Activation and Proinflammatory State in Post-Coronavirus Disease 2019 Syndrome," *Journal of Infectious Diseases* 225, no. 12 (2022): 2155–62; M. Votto et al., "COVID-19 and Autoimmune Diseases: Is There a Connection?," *Current Opinion in Allergy and Clinical Immunology* 23, no. 2 (April 1, 2023): 185–92; R. Chang et al., "Risk of Autoimmune Diseases in Patients with COVID-19: A Retrospective Cohort Study," *eClinicalMedicine* 56 (2023): 101783.

4. NR Rose, "Prediction and Prevention of Autoimmune Disease in the 21st Century: A Review and Preview," *American Journal of Epidemiology* 183, no. 5 (2016): 403–6.

5. L. Wang et al., "Human Autoimmune Diseases: A Comprehensive Update," *Journal of Internal Medicine* 278, no. 4 (2015): 369–95; D. Ray et al., "Immune Senescence, Epigenetics and Autoimmunity," *Clinical Immunology* 196 (2018): 59–63; H. Song et al., "Association of Stress-Related Disorders with Subsequent Autoimmune Disease," *JAMA* 319, no. 23 (2018): 2388–400; M. Mittelbrunn et al., "Hallmarks of T Cell Aging," *Nature Immunology* 22, no. 6 (2021): 687–98; V. Tedeschi et al., "CD8+ T Cell Senescence: Lights and Shadows in Viral Infections, Autoimmune Disorders and Cancer," *International Journal of Molecular Sciences* 23, no. 6 (2022): 3374.

6. DP Bogdanos et al., "Twin Studies in Autoimmune Disease: Genetics, Gender and Environment," *Journal of Autoimmunity* 38, no. 2–3 (2012): J156–69; L. Wang et al., "Human Autoimmune Diseases: A Comprehensive Update," *Journal of Internal Medicine* 278, no. 4 (2015): 369–95; J. Ilonen et al., "The Heterogeneous Pathogenesis of Type 1 Diabetes Mellitus," *Nature Reviews Endocrinology* 15, no. 11 (2019): 635–50.

7. MK Desai et al., "Autoimmune Disease in Women: Endocrine Transition and Risk Across the Lifespan," *Frontiers in Endocrinology* 10, no. 265 (2019); J. Baillargeon et al., "Hypogonadism and the Risk of Rheumatic Autoimmune Disease," *Clinical Rheumatology* 35, no. 12 (2016): 2983–87; R. Bove et al., "Hormones and MS: Risk factors, Biomarkers, and Therapeutic Targets," *Multiple Sclerosis* 24, no. 1 (2018): 17–21.

8. Autoimmune Registry, Inc., 2016–2020, https://www.autoimmuneregistry.org/autoimmune-diseases.

9. V. Martinelli, "Trauma, Stress and Multiple Sclerosis," *Neurological Sciences: Official Journal of the Italian Neurological Society and of the Italian Society of Clinical Neurophysiology* 21, no. 4 (2000): S849–52; M. Cutolo et al., "Stress as a Risk Factor in the Pathogenesis of Rheumatoid

Arthritis," *Neuroimmunomodulation* 13, no. 5–6 (2006): 277–82;
L. Stojanovich et al., "Stress as a Trigger of Autoimmune Disease,"
Autoimmunity Reviews 7, no. 3 (2008): 209–13; MJ McGeachy et al.,
"The IL-17 Family of Cytokines in Health and Disease," *Immunity* 50,
no. 4 (2019): 892–906.

10. J. Brite et al., "The Relationship Between 9/11 Exposure, Systemic
Autoimmune Disease, and Post-Traumatic Stress Disorder: A
Mediational Analysis," *International Journal of Environmental Research
and Public Health* 19, no. 11 (2022): 6514.

11. DB Bookwalter et al., "Posttraumatic Stress Disorder and Risk of
Selected Autoimmune Diseases Among US Military Personnel," *BMC
Psychiatry* 20, no. 1 (2020): 1–8.

12. J. Cookson et al., "Treatment Benefits of Duloxetine in Major
Depressive Disorder as Assessed by Number Needed to Treat,"
International Clinical Psychopharmacology 21, no. 5 (2006): 267–73;
NJ Schork, "Personalized Medicine: Time for One-Person Trials,"
Nature 520, no. 7549 (2015): 609–11; L. Citrome, "Vortioxetine for
Major Depressive Disorder: An Indirect Comparison with Duloxetine,
Escitalopram, Levomilnacipran, Sertraline, Venlafaxine, and Vilazodone,
Using Number Needed to Treat, Number Needed to Harm, and
Likelihood to Be Helped or Harmed," *Journal of Affective Disorders* 196
(2016): 225–33.

13. S. Liang et al., "Recognizing Depression from the Microbiota-Gut-
Brain Axis," *International Journal of Molecular Sciences* 19, no. 6 (2018):
1592; E. Beurel et al., "The Bidirectional Relationship of Depression and
Inflammation: Double Trouble," *Neuron* 107, no. 2 (2020): 234–56; L.
Rudzki et al., "The Microbiota-Gut-Immune-Glia (MGIG) Axis in Major
Depression," *Molecular Neurobiology* 57, no. 10 (2020): 4269–95; R.
Troubat et al., "Neuroinflammation and Depression: A Review," *European
Journal of Neuroscience* 53, no. 1 (2021): 151–71; WC Drevets et al.,
"Immune Targets for Therapeutic Development in Depression: Towards
Precision Medicine," *Nature Reviews Drug Discovery* 21, no. 3 (2022):
224–44; MA Nettis et al., "Is There Neuroinflammation in Depression?
Understanding the Link Between the Brain and the Peripheral Immune
System in Depression," *International Review of Neurobiology* 152 (2020):
23–40, H. Wang et al., "Microglia in Depression: An Overview of
Microglia in the Pathogenesis and Treatment of Depression," *Journal of
Neuroinflammation* 19, no. 1 (2022): 132.

14. C. Williams, "Is Depression a Kind of Allergic Reaction?," *The
Guardian*, January 4, 2015, https://www.theguardian.com/
lifeandstyle/2015/jan/04/depression-allergic-reaction-inflammation-
immune-system.

15. E. Barry, "The 'Nation's Psychiatrist' Takes Stock, with Frustration," *New York Times*, February 2, 2022, https://www.nytimes.com/2022/02/22/us/thomas-insel-book.html.

16. R. Rosmond et al., "The Hypothalamic-Pituitary-Adrenal Axis Activity as a Predictor of Cardiovascular Disease, Type 2 Diabetes and Stroke," *Journal of Internal Medicine* 247, no. 2 (2000): 188–97; BL Bonaz et al., "Brain-Gut Interactions in Inflammatory Bowel Disease," *Gastroenterology* 144, no. 1 (2013): 36–49; B. Brzozowski et al., "Mechanisms by Which Stress Affects the Experimental and Clinical Inflammatory Bowel Disease (IBD): Role of Brain-Gut Axis," *Current Neuropharmacology* 14, no. 8 (2016): 892–900; S. Pellissier et al., "The Place of Stress and Emotions in the Irritable Bowel Syndrome," *Vitamins and Hormones* 103 (2017): 327–54; JJ Joseph et al., "Cortisol Dysregulation: The Bidirectional Link Between Stress, Depression, and Type 2 Diabetes Mellitus," *Annals of the New York Academy of Sciences* 1391, no. 1 (2017): 20–34; VK Sharma et al., "Chronic Stress and Diabetes Mellitus: Interwoven Pathologies," *Current Diabetes Reviews* 16, no. 6 (2020): 546–56; SV Seal et al., "The 'Jekyll and Hyde' of Gluconeogenesis: Early Life Adversity, Later Life Stress, and Metabolic Disturbances," *International Journal of Molecular Sciences* 22, no. 7 (2021): 3344; DN Mishra, "Stress Etiology of Type 2 Diabetes," *Current Diabetes Reviews* 18, no. 9 (2022): e240222201413.

17. T. Mizokami et al., "Stress and Thyroid Autoimmunity," *Thyroid: Official Journal of the American Thyroid Association* 14, no. 12 (2004): 1047–55; MS Harbuz et al., "Stress in Autoimmune Disease Models," *Annals of the New York Academy of Sciences* 1069 (2006): 51–61; R. Geenen et al., "The Impact of Stressors on Health Status and Hypothalamic-Pituitary-Adrenal Axis and Autonomic Nervous System Responsiveness in Rheumatoid Arthritis," *Annals of the New York Academy of Sciences* 1069 (2006): 77–97; M. Cutolo et al., "Stress as a Risk Factor in the Pathogenesis of Rheumatoid Arthritis," *Neuroimmunomodulation* 13, no. 5–6 (2006): 277–82; E. Woźniak et al., "Psychological Stress, Mast Cells, and Psoriasis—Is There Any Relationship?," *International Journal of Molecular Sciences* 22, no. 24 (2021): 13252.

18. G. Weinstein et al., "Glucose Indices Are Associated with Cognitive and Structural Brain Measures in Young Adults," *Neurology* 84, no. 23 (2015): 2329–37; Q. Qianwen et al., "Serum Cortisol Is Associated with Cerebral Small Vessel Disease-Related Brain Changes and Cognitive Impairment," *Frontiers in Aging Neuroscience* 13 (2022): 809684.

19. JB Echouffo-Tcheugui et al., "Circulating Cortisol and Cognitive and Structural Brain Measures: The Framingham Heart Study," *Neurology* 91, no. 21 (2018): e1961–70.

Chapter 2: Trauma, Hormones, and the Root Cause of Autoimmunity

1. M. Pimentel et al., "Autoimmunity Links Vinculin to the Pathophysiology of Chronic Functional Bowel Changes Following Campylobacter Jejuni Infection in a Rat Model," *Digestive Diseases and Sciences* 60, no. 5 (2015): 1195–205; A. Rezaieet, et al., "Assessment of Anti-vinculin and Anti-cytolethal Distending Toxin B Antibodies in Subtypes of Irritable Bowel Syndrome," *Digestive Diseases and Sciences* 62, no. 6 (2017): 1480–85; NJ Talley et al., "Circulating Anti-cytolethal Distending Toxin B and Anti-vinculin Antibodies as Biomarkers in Community and Healthcare Populations with Functional Dyspepsia and Irritable Bowel Syndrome," *Clinical and Translational Gastroenterology* 10, no. 7 (2019): e00064; A. Vojdani et al., "Reaction of Antibodies to Campylobacter Jejuni and Cytolethal Distending Toxin B with Tissues and Food Antigens," *World Journal of Gastroenterology* 25, no. 9 (2019): 1050–66.

2. S. Nochaiwong et al., "Global Prevalence of Mental Health Issues Among the General Population During the Coronavirus Disease–2019 Pandemic: A Systematic Review and Meta-Analysis," *Scientific Reports* 11, no. 1 (2021): 1–18.

3. TA Mudyanadzo et al., "Irritable Bowel Syndrome and Depression: A Shared Pathogenesis," *Cureus* 10, no. 8 (2018).

4. G. Weinstein et al., "Glucose Indices Are Associated with Cognitive and Structural Brain Measures in Young Adults," *Neurology* 84, no. 23 (2015): 2329–37; L. Guzylack-Piriou et al., "Early Life Exposure to Food Contaminants and Social Stress as Risk Factor for Metabolic Disorders Occurrence?—An Overview," *Biomolecules* 11, no. 5 (2021): 687.

5. C. Wallon et al., "Corticotropin-Releasing Hormone (CRH) Regulates Macromolecular Permeability Via Mast Cells in Normal Human Colonic Biopsies in Vitro," *Gut* 57, no. 1 (2008): 50–58; T. Vanuytsel et al., "Psychological Stress and Corticotropin-Releasing Hormone Increase Intestinal Permeability in Humans by a Mast Cell-Dependent Mechanism," *Gut* 63, no. 8 (2014): 1293–99; Y. Sun et al., "Stress-Induced Corticotropin-Releasing Hormone-Mediated NLRP6 Inflammasome Inhibition and Transmissible Enteritis in Mice," *Gastroenterology* 144, no. 7 (2013): 1478–87.

6. S. Fukudo, "Role of Corticotropin-Releasing Hormone in Irritable Bowel Syndrome and Intestinal Inflammation," *Journal of Gastroenterology* 42, no. 17 (2007): 48–51.

7. A. Michielan et al., "Intestinal Permeability in Inflammatory Bowel Disease: Pathogenesis, Clinical Evaluation, and Therapy of Leaky Gut," *Mediators of Inflammation* (2015): 628157; W. Turpin et al., "Increased

Intestinal Permeability Is Associated with Later Development of Crohn's Disease," *Gastroenterology* 159, no. 6 (2020): 2092–100; S. Zhao et al., "Corticotropin Releasing Hormone Promotes Inflammatory Bowel Disease via Inducing Intestinal Macrophage Autophagy," *Cell Death Discovery* 7, no. 1 (2021): 377.

8. S. Mehandru et al., "The Intestinal Barrier, an Arbitrator Turned Provocateur in IBD," *Nature Reviews Gastroenterology & Hepatology* 18, no. 2 (2021): 83–84.

9. A. Fasano, "Zonulin and Its Regulation of Intestinal Barrier Function: The Biological Door to Inflammation, Autoimmunity, and Cancer," *Physiological Reviews* 91, no. 1 (2011): 151–75; A. Fasano, "Leaky Gut and Autoimmune Diseases," *Clinical Reviews in Allergy & Immunology* 42, no. 1 (2012): 71–78; Craig Sturgeon et al., "Zonulin, a Regulator of Epithelial and Endothelial Barrier Functions, and Its Involvement in Chronic Inflammatory Diseases," *Tissue Barriers* 4, no. 4 (2016): e1251384.; P. D'Avino et al., "An Updated Overview on Celiac Disease: From Immuno-Pathogenesis and Immuno-Genetics to Therapeutic Implications," *Expert Review of Clinical Immunology* 17, no. 3 (2021): 269–84; LK Wood Heickman et al., "Zonulin as a Potential Putative Biomarker of Risk for Shared Type 1 Diabetes and Celiac Disease Autoimmunity," *Diabetes/Metabolism Research and Reviews* 36, no. 5 (2020): e3309; H. Ilchmann-Diounou et al., "Psychological Stress, Intestinal Barrier Dysfunctions, and Autoimmune Disorders: An Overview," *Frontiers in Immunology* 11 (2020): 1823; P. D'Avino et al., "An Updated Overview on Celiac Disease: From Immuno-Pathogenesis and Immuno-Genetics to Therapeutic Implications," *Expert Review of Clinical Immunology* 17, no. 3 (2021): 269–84; MM Leonard et al., "Microbiome Signatures of Progression Toward Celiac Disease Onset in At-Risk Children in a Longitudinal Prospective Cohort Study," *Proceedings of the National Academy of Sciences of the United States of America* 118, no. 29 (2021): e2020322118; J. An et al., "The Role of Intestinal Mucosal Barrier in Autoimmune Disease: A Potential Target," *Frontiers in Immunology* 13 (2022): 871713; NE Kushlinskii et al., "Blood Serum Zonulin in Colorectal Cancer, Autoimmune Bowel Diseases, and Irritable Bowel Syndrome," *Bulletin of Experimental Biology and Medicine* (2022), https://pubmed.ncbi.nlm.nih.gov/35852686/.

10. H. Ilchmann-Diounou et al., "Psychological Stress, Intestinal Barrier Dysfunctions, and Autoimmune Disorders: An Overview," *Frontiers in Immunology* 11 (2020): 1823.

11. SR Brand et al., "The Effect of Maternal PTSD Following in Utero Trauma Exposure on Behavior and Temperament in the 9-Month-Old Infant," *Annals of New York Academic Sciences* 1071 (2006): 454–58.

12. The ten genes that reached genome-wide significance in cases of PTSD compared to controls were as follows: CIRBP, TMSB10, FCGRT, CLIC1, RPS6KB2, HNRNPUL1, ALDOA, NACA, ZNF429, and COPE. S. Marchese et al., "Altered Gene Expression and PTSD Symptom Dimensions in World Trade Center Responders," *Molecular Psychiatry* 27, no. 4 (2022): 2225–46.

13. SH Hankerson et al., "The Intergenerational Impact of Structural Racism and Cumulative Trauma on Depression," *American Journal of Psychiatry* 178, no. 6 (2022): 434–40.

14. H. Song et al., "Association of Stress-Related Disorders with Subsequent Autoimmune Disease," *JAMA* 319, no. 23 (2018): 2388–400.

15. R. Glaser et al., "Stress-Induced Immune Dysfunction: Implications for Health," *Nature Reviews Immunology* 5, no. 3 (2005): 243–51.

16. A. O'Donovan et al., "Elevated Risk for Autoimmune Disorders in Iraq and Afghanistan Veterans with Posttraumatic Stress Disorder," *Biological Psychiatry* 77, no. 4 (2015): 365–74; JA Boscarino, "Posttraumatic Stress Disorder and Physical Illness: Results from Clinical and Epidemiologic Studies," *Annals of the New York Academy of Sciences* 1032, no. 1 (2004): 141–53; JA Boscarino et al., "A Twin Study of the Association Between PTSD Symptoms and Rheumatoid Arthritis," *Psychosomatic Medicine* 72, no. 5 (2010): 481–86.

17. G. Frazzei et al., "Preclinical Autoimmune Disease: A Comparison of Rheumatoid Arthritis, Systemic Lupus Erythematosus, Multiple Sclerosis and Type 1 Diabetes," *Frontiers in Immunology* (2022): 3207.

18. S. Rantapää-Dahlqvist et al., "Antibodies Against Cyclic Citrullinated Peptide and IgA Rheumatoid Factor Predict the Development of Rheumatoid Arthritis," *Arthritis & Rheumatism* 48, no. 10 (2003): 2741–49; MMJ Nielen et al., "Increased Levels of C-Reactive Protein in Serum from Blood Donors Before the Onset of Rheumatoid Arthritis," *Arthritis & Rheumatism* 50, no. 8 (2004): 2423–27; MMJ Nielen et al., "Simultaneous Development of Acute Phase Response and Autoantibodies in Preclinical Rheumatoid Arthritis," *Annals of the Rheumatic Diseases* 65, no. 4 (2006): 535–37; LA Van De Stadt et al., "Prediction Rule for the Development of Arthritis in Seropositive Arthralgia Patients," *Annals of the Rheumatic Diseases* 72, no. 12 (2013): 1920–26.

19. R. Glaser et al., "Stress-Induced Immune Dysfunction: Implications for Health," *Nature Reviews Immunology* 5, no. 3 (2005): 243–51.

20. Ibid.; J. Blechert et al., "Autonomic and Respiratory Characteristics of Posttraumatic Stress Disorder and Panic Disorder," *Psychosomatic Medicine* 69, no. 9 (2007): 935–43.

21. G. Frazzei et al., "Preclinical Autoimmune Disease: A Comparison

of Rheumatoid Arthritis, Systemic Lupus Erythematosus, Multiple Sclerosis and Type 1 Diabetes," *Frontiers in Immunology* (2022): 3207.

22. SC Segerstrom et al., "Psychological Stress and the Human Immune System: A Meta-Analytic Study of 30 Years of Inquiry," *Psychological Bulletin* 130, no. 4 (2004): 601.

23. H. Song et al., "Association of Stress-Related Disorders with Subsequent Autoimmune Disease," *JAMA* 319, no. 23 (2018): 2388–400; R. Glaser et al., "Stress-Induced Immune Dysfunction: Implications for Health," *Nature Reviews Immunology* 5, no. 3 (2005): 243–51; J. Blechert et al., "Autonomic and Respiratory Characteristics of Posttraumatic Stress Disorder and Panic Disorder," *Psychosomatic Medicine* 69, no. 9 (2007): 935–43; SC Segerstrom et al., "Psychological Stress and the Human Immune System: A Meta-Analytic Study of 30 Years of Inquiry," *Psychological Bulletin* 130, no. 4 (2004): 601. Measured immune cell activity, such as T-helper lymphocyte counts, natural killer (NK) cell cytotoxicity, and proliferation to phytohemagglutinin.
    G. Frazzei et al., "Preclinical Autoimmune Disease: A Comparison of Rheumatoid Arthritis, Systemic Lupus Erythematosus, Multiple Sclerosis and Type 1 Diabetes," *Frontiers in Immunology* (2022): 3207. Assessed circulating antibodies; inflammatory markers such as high-sensitivity CRP; low omega-3 fatty acid status; and cytokines associated with 5-HETE, such as IL1b, IL-6, IL-8, and TNF.

24. MK Desai et al., "Autoimmune Disease in Women: Endocrine Transition and Risk Across the Lifespan," *Frontiers in Endocrinology* 10, no. 265 (2019).

25. H. He et al., "Association of Maternal Autoimmune Diseases with Risk of Mental Disorders in Offspring in Denmark," *JAMA Network Open* 5, no. 4 (2022): e227503.

26. LT Hoyt et al., "Puberty and Perimenopause: Reproductive Transitions and their Implications for Women's Health," *Social Science & Medicine* 132 (2015): 103–12; MK Desai et al., "Autoimmune Disease in Women: Endocrine Transition and Risk Across the Lifespan," *Frontiers in Endocrinology* 10, no. 265 (2019), HP Priyanka et al., "Neuroimmunomodulation by Estrogen in Health and Disease," *AIMS Neuroscience* 7, no. 4 (2020): 401; A. Mishra et al., "A Tale of Two Systems: Lessons Learned from Female Mid-life Aging with Implications for Alzheimer's Prevention & Treatment," *Ageing Research Reviews* (2021): 101542.

27. HP Priyanka et al., "Neuroimmunomodulation by Estrogen in Health and Disease," *AIMS Neuroscience* 7, no. 4 (2020): 401; A. Mishra et al., "A Tale of Two Systems: Lessons Learned from Female Mid-life Aging

with Implications for Alzheimer's Prevention & Treatment," *Ageing Research Reviews* (2021): 101542.

28. N. Koloski et al., "Population Based Study: Atopy and Autoimmune Diseases Are Associated with Functional Dyspepsia and Irritable Bowel Syndrome, Independent of Psychological Distress," *Alimentary Pharmacology & Therapeutics* 49, no. 5 (2019): 546–55.

29. SH Park et al., "Adverse Childhood Experiences Are Associated with Irritable Bowel Syndrome and Gastrointestinal Symptom Severity," *Neurogastroenterology and Motility: The Official Journal of the European Gastrointestinal Motility Society* 28, no. 8 (2016): 1252–60.

30. H. Rahal et al., "Importance of Trauma-Related Fear in Patients with Irritable Bowel Syndrome and Early Adverse Life Events," *Neurogastroenterology and Motility: The Official Journal of the European Gastrointestinal Motility Society* 32, no. 9 (2020): e13896.

31. T. Ju et al., "Risk and Protective Factors Related to Early Adverse Life Events in Irritable Bowel Syndrome," *Journal of Clinical Gastroenterology* 54, no. 1 (2020): 63–69.

32. C. Mavrangelos et al., "Longitudinal Analysis Indicates Symptom Severity Influences Immune Profile in Irritable Bowel Syndrome," *Gut* 67, no. 2 (2018): 398–99.

33. TA Mudyanadzo et al., "Irritable Bowel Syndrome and Depression: A Shared Pathogenesis," *Cureus* 10, no. 8 (2018); L. Wilmes et al., "Of Bowels, Brain and Behavior: A Role for the Gut Microbiota in Psychiatric Comorbidities in Irritable Bowel Syndrome," *Neurogastroenterology and Motility: The Official Journal of the European Gastrointestinal Motility Society* 33, no. 3 (2021): e14095; MN Aziz et al., "Irritable Bowel Syndrome, Depression, and Neurodegeneration: A Bidirectional Communication from Gut to Brain," *Nutrients* 13, no. 9 (2021): 3061; XF Chen et al., "Aberrant Intraregional Brain Activity and Functional Connectivity in Patients with Diarrhea-Predominant Irritable Bowel Syndrome," *Frontiers in Neuroscience* 15 (2021): 1112.

34. A. Miller, *The Drama of the Gifted Child* (New York: Basic Books, 1979).

35. M. Pluess, "Individual Differences in Environmental Sensitivity," *Child Development Perspectives* 9, no. 3 (2015): 138–43.

36. E. Assary et al., "Genetic Architecture of Environmental Sensitivity Reflects Multiple Heritable Components: A Twin Study with Adolescents," *Molecular Psychiatry* 26, no. 9 (2021): 4896–904.

37. MS Kurcinka, *Raising Your Spirited Child* (New York: William Morrow, 2006).

38. M. Pluess et al., "Environmental Sensitivity in Children: Development of the Highly Sensitive Child Scale and Identification of Sensitivity Groups," *Developmental Psychology* 54, no. 1 (2018): 51.

39. BJ Ellis et al., "Differential Susceptibility to the Environment: Toward an Understanding of Sensitivity to Developmental Experiences and Context," *Development and Psychopathology* 23, no. 1 (2011): 1–5.

40. J. Chow et al., "Pathobionts of the Gastrointestinal Microbiota and Inflammatory Disease," *Current Opinion in Immunology* 23, no. 4 (2011): 473–80; J. Scher et al., "Expansion of Intestinal Prevotella Corpi Relates with Enhanced Susceptibility to Arthritis," *eLife* (2013): 2; C. Zárate-Bladés et al., "Regulation of Autoimmunity by the Microbiome," *DNA and Cell Biology* 35, no. 9 (2016): 455–58; MA Conlon et al., "The Impact of Diet and Lifestyle on Gut Microbiota and Human Health," *Nutrients* 7, no. 1 (2015): 17–44; P. Turnbaugh et al., "Diet-Induced Obesity Is Linked to Marked but Reversible Alterations in the Mouse Distal Gut Microbiome," *Cell Host & Microbe* 3, no. 4 (2008): 213–23; JG Barin et al., "The Microbiome and Autoimmune Disease: Report from a Noel R. Rose Colloquium," *Clinical Immunology* 159, no. 2 (2015): 183–88; GL de Oliveira et al., "Intestinal Dysbiosis in Inflammatory Diseases," *Frontiers in Immunology* 12 (2021).

41. E. Montero-López et al., "Analyses of Hair and Salivary Cortisol for Evaluating Hypothalamic-Pituitary-Adrenal Axis Activation in Patients with Autoimmune Disease," *Stress* 20, no. 6 (2017): 541–48.

42. R. Willemsen et al., "Alexithymia and Dermatology: The State of the Art," *International Journal of Dermatology* 47, no. 9 (2008): 903–10.

43. J. Masmoudi et al., "Alexithymie et Psoriasis: Étude Cas-Témoin à Propos de 53 Patients" [Alexithymia and Psoriasis: A Case-Control Study of 53 Patients], *L'Encephale* 35, no. 1 (2009): 10–17.

44. G. Martino et al., "Alexithymia, Emotional Distress, and Perceived Quality of Life in Patients with Hashimoto's Thyroiditis," *Frontiers in Psychology* 12 (2021): 1295.

45. M. Chimenti et al. "Evaluation of Alexithymia in Patients Affected by Rheumatoid Arthritis and Psoriatic Arthritis: A Cross-Sectional Study," *Medicine* 98, no. 4 (2019): e13955.

46. R. Teggi et al., "Alexithymia in Patients with Ménière Disease: A Possible Role on Anxiety and Depression," *Audiology Research* 11, no. 1 (2021): 63–72.

47. MM Macarenco et al., "Childhood Trauma, Dissociation, Alexithymia, and Anger in People with Autoimmune Diseases: A Mediation Model," *Child Abuse & Neglect* 122 (2021): 105322.

48. M. Gabor, *In the Realm of Hungry Ghosts: Close Encounters with Addiction* (New York: Random House Digital, 2008).

Chapter 3: Understanding Autoimmunity Triggered by Trauma

1. Personal communication with Arielle Schwartz, PhD, by Sara

Gottfried, MD, on May 29, 2023, via email. Learn more at https://drarielleschwartz.com/, accessed May 30, 2023.

2. To learn more, consider Bruce Lipton's book, *The Biology of Belief 10th Anniversary Edition: Unleashing the Power of Consciousness, Matter & Miracles* (Carlsbad, CA: Hay House, Inc. 2016).

3. L. Tolstoy, *Anna Karenina* (New York: Penguin Books, 2016).

4. VJ Felitti et al., "Relationship of Childhood Abuse and Household Dysfunction to Many of the Leading Causes of Death in Adults: The Adverse Childhood Experiences (ACE) Study," *American Journal of Preventive Medicine* 14, no. 4 (1998): 245–58.

5. VJ Felitti et al., "The Relation Between Adverse Childhood Experiences and Adult Health: Turning Gold into Lead," *Permanente Journal* 6, no. 1 (2002): 44–47.

6. AA Akamine et al., "Adverse Childhood Experience in Patients with Psoriasis," *Trends in Psychiatry and Psychotherapy* (2021).

7. DA Drossman et al., "Sexual and Physical Abuse and Gastrointestinal Illness. Review and Recommendations." *Annals of Internal Medicine* 123, no. 10 (1995): 782–94; JE Videlock et al., "Childhood Trauma Is Associated with Hypothalamic-Pituitary-Adrenal Axis Responsiveness in Irritable Bowel Syndrome," *Gastroenterology* 137, no. 6 (2009): 1954–62; K. Bradford et al., "Association Between Early Adverse Life Events and Irritable Bowel Syndrome," *Clinical Gastroenterology and Hepatology: The Official Clinical Practice Journal of the American Gastroenterological Association* 10, no. 4 (2012): 385–90; M. Halland et al., "A Case-control Study of Childhood Trauma in the Development of Irritable Bowel Syndrome," *Neurogastroenterology and Motility: The Official Journal of the European Gastrointestinal Motility Society* 26, no. 7 (2014): 990–98; SH Park et al., "Adverse Childhood Experiences Are Associated with Irritable Bowel Syndrome and Gastrointestinal Symptom Severity," *Neurogastroenterology and Motility: The Official Journal of the European Gastrointestinal Motility Society* 28, no. 8 (2016): 1252–60; JD Rosenblat et al., "Association of History of Adverse Childhood Experiences with Irritable Bowel Syndrome (IBS) in Individuals with Mood Disorders," *Psychiatry Research* 288 (2020): 112967; T. Ju et al., "Risk and Protective Factors Related to Early Adverse Life Events in Irritable Bowel Syndrome," *Journal of Clinical Gastroenterology* 54, no. 1 (2020): 63–69.

8. J. Shreeya et al., "Meta-Analysis and Systematic Review of the Association Between Adverse Childhood Events and Irritable Bowel Syndrome," *Journal of Investigative Medicine: The Official Publication of the American Federation for Clinical Research* 70, no. 6 (2022): 1342–51.

9. NJ Talley et al., "Gastrointestinal Tract Symptoms and Self-reported

Abuse: A Population-Based Study," *Gastroenterology* 107, no. 4 (1994): 1040–49.

10. F. Olivieri et al., "Sex/Gender-Related Differences in Inflammaging." *Mechanisms of Ageing and Development* 211 (2023):111792; RAJ Miller et al. (2023). "Sex Chromosome Complement and Sex Steroid Signaling Underlie Sex Differences in Immunity to Respiratory Virus Infection," *Frontiers in Pharmacology* 14 (2023): 1150282; F. Sciarra et al., "Gender-Specific Impact of Sex Hormones on the Immune System," *International Journal of Molecular Sciences* 24, no. 7 (2023): 6302.

11. HL Köhling et al., "The Microbiota and Autoimmunity: Their Role in Thyroid Autoimmune Diseases," *Clinical Immunology* 183 (2017): 63–74; SK Shukla et al., "Infections, Genetic and Environmental Factors in Pathogenesis of Autoimmune Thyroid Diseases," *Microbial Pathogenesis* 116 (2018): 279–88; M. Zangiabadian et al., "Associations of Yersinia Enterocolitica Infection with Autoimmune Thyroid Diseases: A Systematic Review and Meta-Analysis," *Endocrine, Metabolic & Immune Disorders—Drug Targets* 21, no. 4 (2021): 682–87.

12. R. Yehuda et al., "Gene Expression Patterns Associated with Posttraumatic Stress Disorder Following Exposure to the World Trade Center Attacks," *Biological Psychiatry* 66, no. 7 (2009): 708–11.

13. R. Yehuda et al., "Transgenerational Effects of Posttraumatic Stress Disorder in Babies of Mothers Exposed to the World Trade Center Attacks During Pregnancy." *Journal of Clinical Endocrinology and Metabolism* 90, no. 7 (2005): 4115–4118; R. Yehuda et al., "Gene Expression Patterns Associated with Posttraumatic Stress Disorder Following Exposure to the World Trade Center Attacks," *Biological Psychiatry* 66, no. 7 (2009): 708–11.

14. SR Brand et al., "The Effect of Maternal PTSD Following in Utero Trauma Exposure on Behavior and Temperament in the 9-Month-Old Infant," *Annals of the New York Academy of Sciences* 1071 (2006): 454–58.

Chapter 4: Trauma Is Different for Men and Women

1. Before the pandemic, the World Health Organization performed a survey in twenty-four countries of nearly seventy thousand people and found that 70 percent of respondents experienced serious lifetime traumas, with an average of 3.2 traumas per capita. They concluded that lifetime trauma exposure is so common that it has become the norm for most of us. RC Kessler et al., "Trauma and PTSD in the WHO World Mental Health Surveys," *European Journal of Psychotraumatology* 8, supp. 5 (2017): 1353383.

2. I am committed to inclusivity when writing about sex, bodies, and hormones. I will use sex- and gender-neutral terms when appropriate (e.g., persons) though that's not how research has been done or reported, leading to a challenging gap in this chapter. In general, I am referring to sex assigned at birth in chapter, meaning assigned male at birth or assigned female at birth.
   Guidelines for the Primary and Gender-Affirming Care of Transgender and Gender Nonbinary People, UCSF, 2016. Aaron B. Caughey et al., "USPSTF Approach to Addressing Sex and Gender when Making Recommendations for Clinical Preventive Services," *JAMA* 19, vol. 326 (2021): 1953–61.

3. AJ Bassett et al., "The Biology of Sex and Sport," *JBJS Reviews* 8, no. 3 (2020): e0140.

4. S. Gottfried, *Women, Food and Hormones* (New York: HarperCollins, 2021).

5. R. Lepers, "Sex Difference in Triathlon Performance," *Frontiers in Physiology* 10, no. 973 (2019).

6. DF Tolin et al., "Sex Differences in Trauma and Posttraumatic Stress Disorder: A Quantitative Review of 25 Years of Research," *Psychological Bulletin* 132, no. 6 (2006): 959–92.

7. M. Olff, "Sex and Gender Differences in Post-Traumatic Stress Disorder: An Update," *European Journal of Psychotraumatology* 8, no. 4 (2017): 1351204.

8. ER Palser et al., "Gender and Geographical Disparity in Editorial Boards of Journals in Psychology and Neuroscience," *Nature Neuroscience* 25, no. 3 (2022): 272–79.

9. E. Wolf et al., "The Dissociative Subtype of PTSD Scale: Initial Evaluation in a National Sample of Trauma-Exposed Veterans," *Assessment* 24, no. 4 (2017): 503–16; M. Hansen et al., "Evidence of the Dissociative PTSD Subtype: A Systematic Literature Review of Latent Class and Profile Analytic Studies of PTSD," *Journal of Affective Disorders* 213 (2017): 59–69.

10. PH Taha et al., "Gender Differences in Traumatic Experiences, PTSD, and Relevant Symptoms Among the Iraqi Internally Displaced Persons," *International Journal of Environmental Research and Public Health* 18, no. 18 (2021): 9779.
    As you will learn in later chapters, oxytocin administration is being used to treat PTSD. It's a novel treatment that we will address in this book. JL Frijling, "Preventing PTSD with Oxytocin: Effects of Oxytocin Administration on Fear Neurocircuitry and PTSD Symptom Development in Recently Trauma-Exposed Individuals," *European Journal of Psychotraumatology* 8, no. 1 (2017): 13026516.

11. DF Tolin et al., "Sex Differences in Trauma and Posttraumatic
Stress Disorder: A Quantitative Review of 25 Years of Research,"
Psychological Bulletin 132, no. 6 (2006): 959–92; M. Olff et al., "Gender
Differences in Posttraumatic Stress Disorder," *Psychological Bulletin*
133 no. 2 (2007): 183–204; M. Olff, "Sex and Gender Differences
in Post-Traumatic Stress Disorder: An Update," *European Journal of
Psychotraumatology* 8, no. 4 (2017): 1351204; H. Javidi et al., "Post-
traumatic Stress Disorder," *International Journal of Occupational and
Environmental Medicine* 3, no. 1 (2012): 2–9; R. Kimerling et al.,
"Chromosomes to Social Contexts: Sex and Gender Differences in
PTSD," *Current Psychiatry Reports* 20, no. 12 (2018): 1–9; D Vernor,
"PTSD Is More Likely in Women Than Men," National Alliance on
Mental Illness, October 8, 2019, https://www.nami.org/Blogs/NAMI-
Blog/October-2019/PTSD-is-More-Likely-in-Women-Than-Men; R.
Robles-García et al., Posttraumatic Stress Disorder in Urban Women,"
Current Opinion in Psychiatry 33, no. 3 (2020): 245–49.

12. H. Javidi et al., "Post-traumatic Stress Disorder," *International Journal of
Occupational and Environmental Medicine* 3, no. 1 (2012): 2–9.

13. American Psychological Association, "Facts About Women and Trauma,"
https://www.apa.org/advocacy/interpersonal-violence/women-trauma.

14. M. Olff, "Sex and Gender Differences in Post-Traumatic Stress
Disorder: An Update," *European Journal of Psychotraumatology* 8, no. 4
(2017): 1351204.

15. S. Murphy et al., "Sex Differences in PTSD Symptoms: A Differential
Item Functioning Approach," *Psychological Trauma: Theory, Research,
Practice, and Policy* 11, no. 3 (2019): 319.

16. KT Brady, "Posttraumatic Stress Disorder and Comorbidity:
Recognizing the Many Faces of PTSD," *Journal of Clinical Psychiatry* 58,
no. 9 (1997): 12–15.

17. I. Gardoki-Souto et al., "Prevalence and Characterization of
Psychological Trauma in Patients with Fibromyalgia: A Cross-
Sectional Study," *Pain Research and Management* (2022), doi:
10.1155/2022/2114451.

18. SR Dube et al., "Cumulative Childhood Stress and Autoimmune
Diseases in Adults," *Psychosomatic Medicine* 71, no. 2 (2009): 243.

19. J. Li et al., "The Risk of Multiple Sclerosis in Bereaved Parents: A
Nationwide Cohort Study in Denmark," *Neurology* 62, no. 5 (2004):
726–29.

20. AL Roberts et al., "Posttraumatic Stress Disorder Is Associated with
Increased Risk of Ovarian Cancer: A Prospective and Retrospective
Longitudinal Cohort Study," *Cancer Research* 79, no. 19 (2019):
5113–20.

21. GI Al Jowf et al., "A Public Health Perspective of Post-Traumatic Stress Disorder," *International Journal of Environmental Research and Public Health* 19, no. 11 (2022): 6474.

22. RC Kessler et al., "Trauma and PTSD in the WHO World Mental Health Surveys," *European Journal of Psychotraumatology* 8, supp. 5 (2017): 1353383.

23. M. Olff, "Sex and Gender Differences in Post-Traumatic Stress Disorder: An Update," *European Journal of Psychotraumatology* 8, no. 4 (2017): 1351204.

24. R. Kimerling et al., "Chromosomes to Social Contexts: Sex and Gender Differences in PTSD," *Current Psychiatry Reports* 20, no. 12 (2018): 1–9.

25. AT Geronimus, "The Weathering Hypothesis and the Health of African-American Women and Infants: Evidence and Speculations," *Ethnicity & Disease* (1992): 207–21; AT Geronimus et al., "'Weathering' and Age Patterns of Allostatic Load Scores Among Blacks and Whites in the United States," *American Journal of Public Health* 96, no. 5 (2006): 826–33; KK Schmeer et al., "Racial Ethnic Disparities in Inflammation: Evidence of Weathering in Childhood?," *Journal of Health and Social Behavior* 59, no. 3 (2018): 411–28; S. Forrester et al., "Racial Differences in Weathering and Its Associations with Psychosocial Stress: The CARDIA Study," *SSM-Population Health* 7 (2019): 100319; AT Forde et al., "The Weathering Hypothesis as an Explanation for Racial Disparities in Health: A Systematic Review," *Annals of Epidemiology* 33 (2019): 1–18; AT Geronimus et al., "Weathering, Drugs, and Whack-a-Mole: Fundamental and Proximate Causes of Widening Educational Inequity in U.S. Life Expectancy by Sex and Race, 1990–2015," *Journal of Health and Social Behavior* 60, no. 2 (2019): 222–39; AE Brisendine et al., "The Weathering Hypothesis and Stillbirth: Racial Disparities Across the Life Span," *Ethnicity & Health* 25, no. 3 (2020): 354–66; RL Simons et al., "Racial Discrimination, Inflammation, and Chronic Illness Among African American Women at Midlife: Support for the Weathering Perspective," *Journal of Racial and Ethnic Health Disparities* 8 (2021): 339–49; F. Brewster, "Courage and Fear: Weathering the Collective Racial Storm," *Psychoanalytic Review* 109, no. 1 (2022): 3–12; MD Thomas et al., "Superwoman Schema, Racial Identity, and Cellular Aging Among African American Women," *Gerontologist* 62, no. 5 (2022): 762–72; EM Hailu et al., "Racial/Ethnic Disparities in Severe Maternal Morbidity: An Intersectional Lifecourse Approach," *Annals of the New York Academy of Sciences* (2022), doi: 10.1111/nyas.14901.

26. Refinery29, "How 1,000 Women Feel & Talk About Other People's Bodies—& Their Own," accessed July 19, 2022, https://www.refinery29.com/en-us/women-body-type-positivity-survey.

27. Podcast with Cole Arthur Riley, transcript: https://momastery.com/blog/we-can-do-hard-things-ep-103/ and recording: https://podcasts.apple.com/us/podcast/how-to-be-more-alive-with-cole-arthur-riley/id1564530722?i=1000565730425.

28. Ninety-one percent of rape and sexual assault cases are women, according to the National Sexual Violence Resource Center, "Statistics About Sexual Violence," https://www.nsvrc.org/sites/default/files/publications_nsvrc_factsheet_media-packet_statistics-about-sexual-violence_0.pdf.

29. World Health Organization, "Devastatingly Pervasive: 1 in 3 Women Globally Experience Violence," https://www.who.int/news/item/09-03-2021-devastatingly-pervasive-1-in-3-women-globally-experience-violence.

30. Y. Pan et al., "Prevalence of Childhood Sexual Abuse Among Women Using the Childhood Trauma Questionnaire: A Worldwide Meta-Analysis," *Trauma Violence Abuse* 22, no. 5 (2021): 1181–91.

31. These statistics about rape and sexual abuse are from https://www.rainn.org/resources, accessed August 9, 2022. RAINN is the Rape, Abuse & Incest National Network and is the United States' largest anti–sexual violence organization. From their website: "RAINN created and operates the National Sexual Assault Hotline (800-656-HOPE) in partnership with more than 1,000 local sexual assault serve providers across the country and operates the Department of Defense Safe Helpline."

32. M. Stoltenborgh et al., "A Global Perspective on Child Sexual Abuse: Meta-Analysis of Prevalence Around the World," *Child Maltreatment* 16, no. 2 (2011): 79–101.

33. https://www.rainn.org/resources, accessed August 9, 2022.

34. MJ Breiding, "Prevalence and Characteristics of Sexual Violence, Stalking, and Intimate Partner Violence Victimization—National Intimate Partner and Sexual Violence Survey, United States, 2011," *Morbidity and Mortality Weekly Report. Surveillance Summaries (Washington, DC: 2002)* 63, no. 8 (2014): 1, https://www.cdc.gov/mmwr/preview/mmwrhtml/ss6308a1.htm; L. Sheridan et al., "The Phenomenology of Group Stalking ('Gang-Stalking'): A Content Analysis of Subjective Experiences," *International Journal of Environmental Research and Public Health* 17, no. 7 (2020): 2506; H. Dreßing et al., "The Prevalence and Effects of Stalking: A Replication Study," *Deutsches Ärzteblatt International* 117, no. 20 (2020): 347.

35. C. Benjet et al., "The Epidemiology of Traumatic Event Exposure Worldwide: Results from the World Mental Health Survey Consortium," *Psychological Medicine* 46, no. 2 (2016): 327–43.

36. RC Kessler et al., "Trauma and PTSD in the WHO World Mental Health Surveys," *European Journal of Psychotraumatology* 8, no. supp. 5 (2017): 1353383.

37. M. Olff, "Sex and Gender Differences in Post-Traumatic Stress Disorder: An Update," *European Journal of Psychotraumatology* 8, no. 4 (2017): 1351204.

38. Ibid.

39. TS Ramikie et al., "Mechanisms of Sex Differences in Fear and Posttraumatic Stress Disorder," *Biological Psychiatry* 83, no. 10 (2018): 876–85.

40. C. Carter et al., "Is Oxytocin 'Nature's Medicine'?," *Pharmacological Reviews* 72, no. 4 (2020): 829–61; SR Sharma et al., "What's Love Got to Do With It: Role of Oxytocin in Trauma, Attachment and Resilience," *Pharmacology & Therapeutics* 214 (2020): 107602; MD De Bellis et al., "The Biological Effects of Childhood Trauma," *Child and Adolescent Psychiatric Clinics* 23, no. 2 (2014): 185–222.

41. L. Nawijn et al., "Oxytocin Receptor Gene Methylation in Male and Female PTSD Patients and Trauma-Exposed Controls," *European Neuropsychopharmacology* 29, no. 1 (2019): 147–55; AB Witteveen et al., "The Oxytocinergic System in PTSD Following Traumatic Childbirth: Endogenous and Exogenous Oxytocin in the Peripartum Period," *Archives of Women's Mental Health* 23, no. 3 (2020): 317–29; C. Carmassi et al., "Decreased Plasma Oxytocin Levels in Patients with PTSD," *Frontiers in Psychology* (2021): 1312; J. Hofmann et al., "Oxytocin Receptor Is a Potential Biomarker of the Hyporesponsive HPA Axis Subtype of PTSD and Might be Modulated by HPA Axis Reactivity Traits in Humans and Mice," *Psychoneuroendocrinology* 129 (2021): 105242.

42. M. Olff, "Sex and Gender Differences in Post-Traumatic Stress Disorder: An Update," *European Journal of Psychotraumatology* 8, no. 4 (2017): 1351204.

43. As you will learn in later chapters, oxytocin administration is being used to treat PTSD. It's a novel treatment that we will address in this book. JL Frijling, "Preventing PTSD with Oxytocin: Effects of Oxytocin Administration on Fear Neurocircuitry and PTSD Symptom Development in Recently Trauma-Exposed Individuals," *European Journal of Psychotraumatology* 8, no. 1 (2017): 1302652.

44. M. Olff, "Sex and Gender Differences in Post-Traumatic Stress Disorder: An Update," *European Journal of Psychotraumatology* 8, no. 4 (2017): 1351204.

45. A. Agorastos et al., "Sleep, Circadian System and Traumatic Stress," *European Journal of Psychotraumatology* 12, no. 1 (2021): 1956746.

Chapter 5: Why Pharmaceuticals and Talk Therapy May Not Be Enough

1. G. Vaid et al., "Psychedelic Psychotherapy: Building Wholeness Through Connection," *Global Advances in Health and Medicine* 11 (2022): 2164957X221081113.

2. Now called myalgic encephalomyelitis/chronic fatigue syndrome: https://www.cdc.gov/me-cfs/about/index.html.

3. Department of Veterans Affairs, "VA/DoD Clinical Practice Guideline for the Management of Posttraumatic Stress Disorder and Acute Stress Disorder Pocket Card," https://www.healthquality.va.gov/guidelines/ MH/ptsd/VADoDPTSDCPGPocketCardFinal508-082918b.pdf.

4. JM Mitchell et al., "MDMA-Assisted Therapy for Severe PTSD: A Randomized, Double-Blind, Placebo-Controlled Phase 3 Study," *Nature Medicine* 27, (2021): 1025–33.

5. J. Elflein, "Percentage of U.S. Adults Aged 18 Years and Older Who Had Received Any Mental Health Treatment or Medication in the Past 12 Months in 2020, by Gender," October 29, 2021, https://www .statista.com/statistics/1193044/share-adults-who-received-any-mental-health-treatment-medication-by-gender-us. These data are consistent with data from the Centers for Disease Control and Prevention, and the National Center for Health Statistics. A. Petersen, "Why So Many Women in Middle Age Are on Antidepressants," April 2, 2022, https:// www.wsj.com/articles/why-so-many-middle-aged-women-are-on-antidepressants-11648906393.

6. J. Elflein, "Percentage of U.S. Adults Aged 18 Years and Older Who Had Received Any Mental Health Treatment or Medication in the Past 12 Months in 2020, by Gender," October 29, 2021, https://www .statista.com/statistics/1193044/share-adults-who-received-any-mental-health-treatment-medication-by-gender-us.

7. V. Bekiempis, "Why One in Four Women Is on Psych Meds," *The Guardian,* November 21, 2011, https://www.theguardian.com/ commentisfree/cifamerica/2011/nov/21/one-in-four-women-psych-meds; S. Roan, "One in Five U.S. Adults Takes Medication for a Mental Disorder," *Los Angeles Times*, November 16, 2011, https://www.latimes .com/health/la-xpm-2011-nov-16-la-heb-mental-health-20111116-story .html; LA Pratt et al., "Antidepressant Use Among Persons Aged 12 and Over: United States, 2011–2014," August 2017, https://www.cdc.gov/ nchs/products/databriefs/db283.htm.

8. DJ Brody et al., "Antidepressant Use Among Adults: United States, 2015–2018," September 2020, https://www.cdc.gov/nchs/products/ databriefs/db377.htm.

9. JI Bisson et al., "Prevention and Treatment of PTSD: The Current

Evidence Base," *European Journal of Psychotraumatology* 12, no. 1 (2021): 1824381.

10. "Selective serotonin reuptake inhibitors (SSRIs) were found to be statistically superior to placebo in reduction of PTSD symptoms but the effect size was small (standardised mean difference –0.28, 95% CI –0.39 to –0.17). For individual monotherapy agents compared to placebo in two or more studies, we found small statistically significant evidence for the antidepressants fluoxetine, paroxetine, sertraline, venlafaxine and the antipsychotic quetiapine. For pharmacological augmentation, we found small statistically significant evidence for prazosin and risperidone." MD Hoskins et al., "Pharmacological Therapy for Post-traumatic Stress Disorder: A Systematic Review and Meta-Analysis of Monotherapy, Augmentation and Head-to-Head Approaches," *European Journal of Psychotraumatology* 12, no. 1 (2021): 1802920.

11. Ibid.; M. Jeffreys, "Clinician's Guide to Medications for PTSD," PTSD: National Center for PTSD, https://www.ptsd.va.gov/professional/treat/txessentials/clinician_guide_meds.asp#top.

12. B. Arroll et al., "Antidepressants Versus Placebo for Depression in Primary Care," *Cochrane Database of Systematic Reviews* 3 (2009): CD007954.

13. I. Kirsch et al., "Listening to Prozac but Hearing Placebo: A Meta-Analysis of Antidepressant Medication," *Prevention & Treatment* 1, no. 2 (2019); J. Bacaltchuk et al., "Antidepressants Versus Psychological Treatments and Their Combination for Bulimia Nervosa," *Cochrane Database of Systematic Reviews* 4 (2001); M. Sinyor et al., "The Sequenced Treatment Alternatives to Relieve Depression (STAR*D) Trial: A Review," *Canadian Journal of Psychiatry* 55, no. 3 (2010): 126–35; W. Häuser et al., "The Role of Antidepressants in the Management of Fibromyalgia Syndrome: A Systematic Review and Meta-Analysis," *CNS Drugs* 26, no. 4 (2012): 297–307; A. Tham et al., "Efficacy and Tolerability of Antidepressants in People Aged 65 Years or Older with Major Depressive Disorder—A Systematic Review and a Meta-Analysis," *Journal of Affective Disorders* 205 (2016): 1–12; B. Arroll et al., "Antidepressants for Treatment of Depression in Primary Care: A Systematic Review and Meta-Analysis," *Journal of Primary Health Care* 8, no. 4 (2016): 325–34; AJ Rush et al., "Clinical Implications of the STAR*D Trial," *Handbook of Experimental Pharmacology* 250 (2019): 51–99.

14. "Methotrexate monotherapy showed a clinically important and statistically significant improvement in the American College of Rheumatology 50 response rate when compared with placebo at

52 weeks" with a number needed to treat (NNT) "7, (95% confidence interval 4 to 22)." MA Lopez-Olivo et al., "Methotrexate for Treating Rheumatoid Arthritis," *Cochrane Database of Systematic Reviews* 6 (2014).

15. "Rituximab is a selective, B-cell depleting, biologic agent for treating refractory rheumatoid arthritis (RA). It is a chimeric monoclonal antibody targeted against CD 20 that is promoted as therapy for patients who fail to respond to other biologics." It is usually given with methotrexate. MA Lopez-Olivo et al., "Rituximab for Rheumatoid Arthritis," *Cochrane Database of Systematic Reviews* 1 (2015).

16. LE Kristensen et al., "The Number Needed to Treat for Second-Generation Biologics When Treating Established Rheumatoid Arthritis: A Systematic Quantitative Review of Randomized Controlled Trials," *Scandinavian Journal of Rheumatology* 40, no. 1 (2011): 1–7.

17. A. Pierreisnard et al., "Meta-Analysis of Clinical and Radiological Efficacy of Biologics in Rheumatoid Arthritis Patients Naive or Inadequately Responsive to Methotrexate," *Joint Bone Spine* 80, no. 4 (2013): 386–92.

18. TF Galvao et al., "Withdrawal of Biologic Agents in Rheumatoid Arthritis: A Systematic Review and Meta-Analysis," *Clinical Rheumatology* 35, no. 7 (2016): 1659–68.

19. Immune suppressants are used for people with autoimmune disease, as well as for people who've had an organ transplant. DB Herrmann et al., "Drugs in Autoimmune Diseases," *Klinische Wochenschrift* 68 (1990): 15–25; PJ Eggenhuizen et al., "Treg Enhancing Therapies to Treat Autoimmune Diseases," *International Journal of Molecular Sciences* 21, no. 19 (2020): 7015; M. Meneghini et al., "Immunosuppressive Drugs Modes of Action," *Best Practice & Research Clinical Gastroenterology* 54 (2021): 101757; G. Handley et al., "Adverse Effects of Immunosuppression: Infections," *Handbook of Experimental Pharmacology* 272 (2022): 287–314; A. Tison et al., "Immune-Checkpoint Inhibitor Use in Patients with Cancer and Pre-existing Autoimmune Diseases," *Nature Reviews Rheumatology* (2022): 1–16.

20. L. Rankin, *Sacred Medicine: A Doctor's Quest to Unravel the Mysteries of Healing* (Louisville, CO: Sounds True, 2022), 249.

21. B. van der Kolk, "Trauma, Attachment, and Neuroscience Training," https://catalog.pesi.com/item/trauma-attachment-neuroscience-bessel-van-der-kolk-md-brain-mind-body-healing-trauma-27080.

22. "Eye Movement Desensitization and Reprocessing (EMDR) for PTSD," PTSD: National Center for PTSD, accessed May 30, 2023, https://www.ptsd.va.gov/understand_tx/emdr.asp23.

23. AK Niazi and SK Niazi, "Mindfulness Based Stress Reduction: A Non-pharmacological Approach for Chronic Illnesses," *North American Journal of Medicine and Science* 3, no. 1 (2011): 20–23.

SN Katterman et al., "Mindfulness Meditation as an Intervention for Binge Eating, Emotional Eating, and Weight Loss: A Systematic Review," *Eating Behaviors* 15, no. 2 (2014): 197–204, doi:10.1016/j.eatbeh.2014.01.005.

M. Janssen et al., "Effects of Mindfulness-Based Stress Reduction on Employees' Mental Health: A Systematic Review," *PloS One* 13, no. 1 (January 24, 2018): e0191332, doi:10.1371/journal.pone.0191332.

C. Conversano et al., "Is Mindfulness-Based Stress Reduction Effective for People with Hypertension? A Systematic Review and Meta-Analysis of 30 Years of Evidence," *International Journal of Environmental Research and Public Health* 18, no. 6 (March 11, 2021): 2882, doi:10.3390/ijerph18062882.

V. Fisher, WW Li, and U. Malabu, "The Effectiveness of Mindfulness-Based Stress Reduction (MBSR) on the Mental Health, HbA1C, and Mindfulness of Diabetes Patients: A Systematic Review and Meta-Analysis of Randomised Controlled Trials," *Applied Psychology: Health and Well-Being*, February 28, 2023, doi:10.1111/aphw.12441.

Q. Liu, J. Zhu, and W. Zhang, "The Efficacy of Mindfulness-Based Stress Reduction Intervention 3 for Post-traumatic Stress Disorder (PTSD) Symptoms in Patients with PTSD: A Meta-Analysis of Four Randomized Controlled Trials," *Stress Health* 38, no. 4 (October 2022): 626–36.

24. V. Fisher, WW Li, and U. Malabu, "The Effectiveness of Mindfulness-Based Stress Reduction (MBSR) on the Mental Health, HbA1C, and Mindfulness of Diabetes Patients: A Systematic Review and Meta-Analysis of Randomised Controlled Trials," *Applied Psychology: Health and Well-Being*, February 28, 2023, doi:10.1111/aphw.12441.

25. A. Kelly and EL Garland, "Trauma-Informed Mindfulness-Based Stress Reduction for Female Survivors of Interpersonal Violence: Results from a Stage I RCT," *Journal of Clinical Psychology* 72, no. 4 (2016): 311–28; AM Gallegos et al., "Effects of Mindfulness Training on Posttraumatic Stress Symptoms from a Community-Based Pilot Clinical Trial Among Survivors of Intimate Partner Violence," *Psychological Trauma* 12, no. 8 (2020): 859–68, epub September 24, 2020, doi:10.1037/tra0000975.

26. MC Mithoefer et al., "MDMA-Assisted Psychotherapy for Treatment of PTSD: Study Design and Rationale for Phase 3 Trials Based on Pooled Analysis of Six Phase 2 Randomized Controlled Trials," *Psychopharmacology* 236 (2019): 2735–45.

27. JM Mitchell et al., "MDMA-Assisted Therapy for Severe PTSD: A Randomized, Double-Blind, Placebo-Controlled Phase 3 Study," *Nature Medicine* 27 (2021): 1025–33.

28. MD Hoskins et al., "Pharmacological Therapy for Post-traumatic Stress Disorder: A Systematic Review and Meta-Analysis of Monotherapy, Augmentation and Head-to-Head Approaches," *European Journal of Psychotraumatology* 12, no. 1 (2021): 1802920.

29. JI Bisson et al., "Evidence-Based Prescribing for Post-traumatic Stress Disorder," *British Journal of Psychiatry* 216, no. 3 (2020): 125–26.

30. JI Bisson et al., "Non-Pharmacological and Non-Psychological Approaches to the Treatment of PTSD: Results of a Systematic Review and Meta-analyses," *European Journal of Psychotraumatology* 11, no. 1 (2020): 1795361.

Chapter 6: Body Awareness

1. N. Piran et al., "The Developmental Theory of Embodiment," *Preventing Eating-Related and Weight-Related Disorders: Collaborative Research, Advocacy, and Policy Change* (2012): 169–98.

2. TL Tylka et al., "The Experience of Embodiment Construct: Reflecting the Quality of Embodied Lives," *Handbook of Positive Body Image and Embodiment: Constructs, Protective Factors, and Interventions* (2019): 11–21.

3. There are many embodiment scales that you can review: Embodied Sense of Self Scale (ESSS), Experiences of Embodiment Scale (EES), the Embodied Mindfulness Scale, Gender Embodiment Scale. These measures vary in their validation and reliability. See also my friend Rachel Carlton Abrams's book *Body Wise*, which I've drawn upon with her permission for the questionnaire in this chapter. R. Carlton Abrams, *Body Wise: Discovering Your Body's Intelligence for Lifelong Health and Healing* (New York: Rodale, 2016); T. Asai et al., "Development of Embodied Sense of Self Scale (ESSS): Exploring Everyday Experiences Induced by Anomalous Self-Representation," *Frontiers in Psychology* 7 (2016): 1005; L. DuBois et al., "Development of the Gender Embodiment Scale: Trans Masculine Spectrum," *Transgender Health* 7, no. 4 (2022): 287–91; B. Khoury et al., "Embodied Mindfulness Questionnaire: Scale Development and Validation," *Assessment* (2021): 10731911211059856; M.R. Longo et al., "What Is Embodiment? A Psychometric Approach," *Cognition* 107, no. 3 (2008): 978–98; N. Piran et al., "The Experience of Embodiment Scale: Development and Psychometric Evaluation," *Body Image* 34 (2020): 117–34.

4. Note that recent experience and discussion with my colleague Omid

Naim, MD, suggests that naltrexone may be helpful as part of a trauma-informed approach to address dissociation.

5. EL Barratt et al., "Autonomous Sensory Meridian Response (ASMR): A Flow-Like Mental State," *PeerJ* 3 (2015): e851; S. Glim et al., "Body Scan Meditation Enhances the Autonomous Sensory Meridian Response to Auditory Stimuli," *Perception* 51, no. 6 (2022): 435–37.

6. HH Ng et al., "Mindfulness Training Associated with Resting-State Electroencephalograms Dynamics in Novice Practitioners *via* Mindful Breathing and Body-Scan," *Frontiers in Psychology* 12 (2021): 748584.

7. F. D'Antoni et al., "Psychotherapeutic Techniques for Distressing Memories: A Comparative Study Between EMDR, Brainspotting, and Body Scan Meditation," *International Journal of Environmental Research and Public Health* 19, no. 3 (2022): 1142. Note that *Brainspotting* is a focused "treatment method that works by identifying, processing and releasing core neurophysiological sources of emotional/body pain, trauma, dissociation and a variety of other challenging symptoms" and will be described more in the next chapter.

8. R. Gan et al., "The Effects of Body Scan Meditation: A Systematic Review and Meta-Analysis, *Applied Psychology: Health and Well-Being* 14, no. 3 (2022): 1062–80.

9. DD Colgan et al., "The Body Scan and Mindful Breathing Among Veterans with PTSD: Type of Intervention Moderates the Relationship Between Changes in Mindfulness and Post-treatment Depression," *Mindfulness* 7, no. 2 (2016): 372–83.

10. M. Ussher et al., "Immediate Effects of a Brief Mindfulness-Based Body Scan on Patients with Chronic Pain," *Journal of Behavioral Medicine* 37, no.1 (2014): 127–34.

11. MJ Goodman et al., "A Mindfulness Course Decreases Burnout and Improves Well-Being Among Healthcare Providers," *International Journal of Psychiatry in Medicine* 43, no. 2 (2012): 119–28.

12. D. Fischer et al., "Improvement of Interoceptive Processes After an 8-Week Body Scan Intervention," *Frontiers in Human Neuroscience* 11 (2017): 452.

13. L. Mirams et al., "Brief Body-Scan Meditation Practice Improves Somatosensory Perceptual Decision Making," *Consciousness and Cognition* 22, no. 1 (2013): 348–59.

14. B. Ditto et al., "Short-Term Autonomic and Cardiovascular Effects of Mindfulness Body Scan Meditation," *Annals of Behavioral Medicine* 32, no. 3 (2006): 227–34.

15. J. Nestor, *Breath: The New Science of a Lost Art* (London: Penguin Life, 2020).

16. DM Eisenberg et al., "Unconventional Medicine in the United States.

Prevalence, Costs, and Patterns of Use," *New England Journal of Medicine* 328, no. 4 (1993): 246–52.

17. S. Grof, "Human Nature and the Nature of Reality: Conceptual Challenges from Consciousness Research," *Journal of Psychoactive Drugs* 30, no. 4 (1998): 343–57.

18. "About Holotropic Breathwork®," http://www.holotropic.com/holotropic-breathwork/about-holotropic-breathwork/.

19. The sitter's role is to be present and available to assist the breather—not to interfere, interrupt, or try to guide the process. Additional elements of the process include focused energy release work and integration practices. Certified facilitators also serve as sitters.

20. JP Rhinewine et al., "Holotropic Breathwork: The Potential Role of a Prolonged, Voluntary Hyperventilation Procedure as an Adjunct to Psychotherapy," *Journal of Alternative and Complementary Medicine* 13, no. 7 (2007): 771–76.

21. P. Shah, "A Primer of the Chakra System," August 20, 2022, https://chopra.com/articles/what-is-a-chakra.

22. BA Brennan, *Hands of Light: A Guide to Healing Through the Human Energy Field* (New York: Bantam, 1987), 71.

23. T. Miller et al., "Measure of Significance of Holotropic Breathwork in the Development of Self-Awareness," *Journal of Alternative and Complementary Medicine* 21, no. 12 (2015): 796–803.

24. S. Grof and C. Grof, *Holotropic Breathwork: A New Approach to Self-Exploration and Therapy* (New York: State University of New York Press, 2010), 7.

25. L. Wisneski et al., "The Scientific Basis of Integrative Medicine," *Evidence-Based Complementary and Alternative Medicine* 2, no. 2 (2005): 257–59.

26. H. Weiss et al., *Hakomi Mindfulness-Centered Somatic Psychotherapy: A Comprehensive Guide to Theory and Practice* (New York: W. W. Norton & Company, 2015), 34–35.

Chapter 7: Testing

1. L. Wang et al., "Human Autoimmune Diseases: A Comprehensive Update," *Journal of Internal Medicine* 278, no. 4 (2015): 369–95.

2. D. Furman et al., "Chronic Inflammation in the Etiology of Disease Across the Life Span," *Nature Medicine* 25, no. 12 (2019): 1822–32.

3. M. Saccucci et al., "Autoimmune Diseases and Their Manifestations on Oral Cavity: Diagnosis and Clinical Management," *Journal of Immunology Research* (2018).

4. CE Wee et al., "Understanding Breast Implant Illness, Before and After Explantation: A Patient-Reported Outcomes Study," *Annals of Plastic*

Surgery 85, S1 suppl. 1 (2020): S82; S. Yang et al., "Understanding Breast Implant Illness: Etiology Is the Key," *Aesthetic Surgery Journal* 42, no. 4 (2022): 370–77; CEE de Vries et al., "Understanding Breast Implant–Associated Illness: A Delphi Survey Defining Most Frequently Associated Symptoms," *Plastic and Reconstructive Surgery* 149, no. 6 (2022): 1056e–61e.

5. Centers for Disease Control and Prevention, "Nearly One in Five American Adults Who Have Had COVID-19 Still Have "Long COVID," accessed December 19, 2022, https://www.cdc.gov/nchs/pressroom/nchs_press_releases/2022/20220622.htm.

6. SE Chang et al., "New-onset IgG Autoantibodies in Hospitalized Patients with COVID-19," *Nature Communications* 12, no. 1 (2021): 1–15.

7. JA James in Workshop on Post-Acute Sequelae of COVID-19, December 4, 2020, https://tracs.unc.edu/index.php/calendar/83-other-sponsor/1766-niaid-workshop-on-covid-19.

8. K. Son et al., "Circulating Anti-nuclear Autoantibodies in COVID-19 Survivors Predict Long-COVID Symptoms," *European Respiratory Journal* (2022).

9. S. Yapeng et al., "Multiple Early Factors Anticipate Post-acute COVID-19 Sequelae," *Cell* 185, no. 5 (2022): 881–95.

10. JA James et al., "Epstein–Barr Virus and Systemic Lupus Erythematosus," *Current Opinion in Rheumatology* 18, no. 5 (2006): 462–67; A. Kaul et al., "Systemic Lupus Erythematosus," *Nature Reviews Disease Primers* 26, no. 2 (2016): 16039; R. Illescas et al., "Infectious Processes and Systemic Lupus Erythematosus," *Immunology* 158, no. 3 (2019): 153–60; G. Houen et al., "Epstein-Barr Virus and Systemic Autoimmune Diseases," *Frontiers in Immunology* 7, no. 11 (2021): 587380; NR Jog et al., "Epstein Barr Virus and Autoimmune Responses in Systemic Lupus Erythematosus," *Frontiers in Immunology* 3, no. 11 (2021): 623944.

11. B. Piccini et al., "Type 1 Diabetes Onset and Pandemic Influenza A (H1N1)," *International Journal of Immunopathology and Pharmacology* 25, no. 2 (2012): 547–49; R. Nenna et al., "Detection of Respiratory Viruses in the 2009 Winter Season in Rome: 2009 Influenza A (H1N1) Complications in Children and Concomitant Type 1 Diabetes Onset," *International Journal of Immunopathology and Pharmacology* 24, no. 3 (2011): 651–59; MK Smatti et al., "Viruses and Autoimmunity: A Review on the Potential Interaction and Molecular Mechanisms," *Viruses* 11, no. 8 (2019): 762; Y. Nishioka et al., "Association Between Influenza and the Incidence Rate of New-Onset Type 1 Diabetes in Japan," *Journal of Diabetes Investigation* 12, no. 10 (2021): 1797–804.

12. PLD Ruiz et al., "Pandemic Influenza and Subsequent Risk of Type 1 Diabetes: A Nationwide Cohort Study," *Diabetologia* 61, no. 9 (2018): 1996–2004.

13. Fulvia Ceccarelli et al., "Genetic Factors of Autoimmune Diseases," *Journal of Immunology Research* 2016 (2016): 3476023, doi:10.1155/2016/3476023.

14. DP Bogdanos et al., "Twin Studies in Autoimmune Disease: Genetics, Gender and Environment," *Journal of Autoimmunity* 38, no. 2–3 (2012): J156–69, doi:10.1016/j.jaut.2011.11.003.

15. An example of a monogenic autoimmune disease is a rare condition called immunodysregulation polyendocrinopathy enteropathy X-linked (IPEX). It primarily affects males and is characterized by immunodeficiency and multi-organ autoimmunity. RS Wildin et al., "Clinical and Molecular Features of the Immunodysregulation, Polyendocrinopathy, Enteropathy, X linked (IPEX) Syndrome," *Journal of Medical Genetics* 39, no. 8 (2002): 537–45; F. Barzaghi et al., "Immune Dysregulation, Polyendocrinopathy, Enteropathy, X-linked Syndrome: A Paradigm of Immunodeficiency with Autoimmunity," *Frontiers in Immunology* 3, no. 211 (2012); M. Jamee et al., "Clinical, Immunological, and Genetic Features in Patients with Immune Dysregulation, Polyendocrinopathy, Enteropathy, X-linked (IPEX) and IPEX-like Syndrome," *Journal of Allergy and Clinical Immunology: In Practice* 8, no. 8 (2020): 2747–60; DT Duztas et al., "New Findings of Immunodysregulation, Polyendocrinopathy, and Enteropathy X-Linked Syndrome (IPEX); Granulomas in Lung and Duodenum," *Pediatric and Developmental Pathology* 24, no. 3 (2021): 252–57.

16. G. Frazzei et al., "Prevention of Rheumatoid Arthritis: A Systematic Literature Review of Preventive Strategies in At-Risk Individuals," *Autoimmunity Reviews* (2022): 103217.

17. P. Du et al., "HLA-DRA Gene Polymorphisms Are Associated with Graves' Disease as an Autoimmune Thyroid Disease," *BioMed Research International* 2022 (2022).

18. "Quantifying Your Body: A How-to Guide from a Systems Biology Perspective," *Biotechnology Journal* 7, no. 8 (2012): 980–91.

19. E. Miyauchi et al., "The Impact of the Gut Microbiome on Extra-intestinal Autoimmune Diseases," *Nature Reviews Immunology* 23, no. 1 (2023): 9–23.

20. D. McDonald et al., "American Gut: An Open Platform for Citizen Science Microbiome Research," *mSystems* 3, no. 3 (2018): e00031-18, https://journals.asm.org/doi/10.1128/msystems.00031-18.

21. L. Smarr et al., "Tracking Human Gut Microbiome Changes Resulting from a Colonoscopy," *Methods of Information in Medicine* 56, no. 6

(2017): 442–47; X. Fang et al., "Metagenomics-Based, Strain-Level Analysis of *Escherichia coli* from a Time-Series of Microbiome Samples from a Crohn's Disease Patient," *Frontiers in Microbiology* 9 (2018): 2559; C. Allaband et al., "Microbiome 101: Studying, Analyzing, and Interpreting Gut Microbiome Data for Clinicians," *Clinical Gastroenterology and Hepatology* 17, no. 2 (2019): 218–30; A. Tripathi et al., "Are Microbiome Studies Ready for Hypothesis-driven Research?," *Current Opinion in Microbiology* 44 (2018): 61–69; X. Fang et al., "Escherichia coli B2 Strains Prevalent in Inflammatory Bowel Disease Patients Have Distinct Metabolic Capabilities that Enable Colonization of Intestinal Mucosa," *BMC Systems Biology* 12 (2018): 1–10; RH Mills et al., "Evaluating Metagenomic Prediction of the Metaproteome in a 4.5-Year Study of a Patient with Crohn's Disease," *mSystems* 4, no. 1 (2019): e00337-18, https://www.ncbi.nlm.nih .gov/pmc/articles/PMC6372841/; Q. Zhu et al., "Phylogenomics of 10,575 Genomes Reveals Evolutionary Proximity Between Domains Bacteria and Archaea," *Nature Communications* 10, no. 1 (2019): 5477; X. Fang et al., "Gastrointestinal Surgery for Inflammatory Bowel Disease Persistently Lowers Microbiome and Metabolome Diversity," *Inflammatory Bowel Diseases* 27, no. 5 (2021): 603–16.

22. F. De Luca et al., "The Microbiome in Autoimmune Diseases," *Clinical and Experimental Immunology* 195, no. 1 (2019): 74–85.

23. The index of microflora richness used in this study of $n = 196$ patients with autoimmune thyroid disease was called Chao1. "Chao1, the index of the microflora richness, was increased in the Hashimoto's thyroiditis group compared to controls (SMD, 0.68, 95%CI: 0.16 to 1.20), while it was decreased in the Graves' disease group (SMD, -0.87, 95%CI: -1.46 to -0.28). In addition, we found that some beneficial bacteria like *Bifidobacterium* and *Lactobacillus* were decreased in the AITD group, and harmful microbiota like *Bacteroides fragilis* was significantly increased compared with the controls." B. Gong et al., "Association Between Gut Microbiota and Autoimmune Thyroid Disease: A Systematic Review and Meta-Analysis," *Frontiers in Endocrinology* (2021): 1544.

24. VB Young et al., "Overview of the Gastrointestinal Microbiota," *Advances in Experimental Medicine and Biology* 635 (2008): 29–40.

25. F. De Luca et al., "The Microbiome in Autoimmune Diseases," *Clinical and Experimental Immunology* 195, no. 1 (2019): 74–85.

26. EA Yamamoto et al., "Between Vitamin D, Gut Microbiome, and Systemic Autoimmunity," *Frontiers in Immunology* 10 (2020): 3141; M. Wolter et al., "Leveraging Diet to Engineer the Gut Microbiome," *Nature Reviews Gastroenterology & Hepatology* 18, no. 12 (2021): 885–902.

27. JA James et al., "Latent Autoimmunity Across Disease-Specific Boundaries in At-Risk First-Degree Relatives of SLE and RA Patients," *eBioMedicine* 42 (2019): 76–85.

28. C. Tani et al., "Rhupus Syndrome: Assessment of Its Prevalence and Its Clinical and Instrumental Characteristics in a Prospective Cohort of 103 SLE Patients," *Autoimmunity Reviews* 12, no. 4 (2013): 537–41.

29. AE Handel et al., "Type 1 Diabetes Mellitus and Multiple Sclerosis: Common Etiological Features," *Nature Reviews Endocrinology* 5, no. 12 (2009): 655–64; P. Tettey et al., "The Co-Occurrence of Multiple Sclerosis and Type 1 Diabetes: Shared Aetiologic Features and Clinical Implication for MS Aetiology," *Journal of the Neurological Sciences* 348, no. 1–2 (2015): 126–31.

30. VL Kronzer et al., "Comorbidities as Risk Factors for Rheumatoid Arthritis and Their Accrual After Diagnosis," *Mayo Clinic Proceedings* 94, no. 12 (2019): 2488–98.

Chapter 8: Nutrition Protocol

1. "Autoimmune Diseases," Prof. Valter Longo, accessed May 30, 2023, https://www.valterlongo.com/autoimmune-diseases/.

2. EA Yamamoto et al., "Relationships Between Vitamin D, Gut Microbiome, and Systemic Autoimmunity," *Frontiers in Immunology* 10 (2020): 3141; M. Wolter et al., "Leveraging Diet to Engineer the Gut Microbiome," *Nature Reviews Gastroenterology & Hepatology* 18, no. 12 (2021): 885–902.

3. KB Hagen et al., "Dietary Interventions for Rheumatoid Arthritis," *Cochrane Database of Systematic Reviews* 1 (2009); SK Tedeschi et al., "Is There a Role for Diet in the Therapy of Rheumatoid Arthritis?," *Current Rheumatology Reports* 18 (2016): 1–9; S. Petersson et al., "The Mediterranean Diet, Fish Oil Supplements and Rheumatoid Arthritis Outcomes: Evidence from Clinical Trials," *Autoimmunity Reviews* 17, no. 11 (2018): 1105–14; J. Nelson et al., "Do Interventions with Diet or Dietary Supplements Reduce the Disease Activity Score in Rheumatoid Arthritis? A Systematic Review of Randomized Controlled Trials," *Nutrients* 12, no. 10 (2020): 2991; E. Philippou et al., "Rheumatoid Arthritis and Dietary Interventions: Systematic Review of Clinical Trials," *Nutrition Reviews* 79, no. 4 (2021): 410–28; Y. Matsumoto et al., "Change in Dietary Inflammatory Index Score Is Associated with Control of Long-Term Rheumatoid Arthritis Disease Activity in a Japanese Cohort: The TOMORROW Study," *Arthritis Research & Therapy* 23, no. 1 (2021): 1–10; M. Lanspa et al., "A Systematic Review of Nutritional Interventions on Key Cytokine Pathways in Rheumatoid Arthritis and Its Implications for Comorbid

Depression: Is a More Comprehensive Approach Required?," *Cureus* 14, no. 8 (2022): e2803; S. Xiang et al., "The Association Between Dietary Inflammation Index and the Risk of Rheumatoid Arthritis in Americans," *Clinical Rheumatology* 41, no. 9 (2022): 2647–58.

4. TL Wahls, "Dietary Approaches to Treating Multiple Sclerosis-Related Symptoms," *Physical Medicine and Rehabilitation Clinics* 33, no. 3 (2022): 605–20.

5. T regulatory cells, also known as Treg, can be induced to support the immune system to a state of balance. B. Prietl et al., "Vitamin D and Immune Function," *Nutrients* 5, no. 7 (2013): 2502–21; MT Cantorna et al., "Vitamin D and 1,25(OH)2D Regulation of T Cells," *Nutrients* 7, no. 4 (2015): 3011–21; Y. Alwarawrah et al., "Changes in Nutritional Status Impact Immune Cell Metabolism and Function," *Frontiers in Immunology* (2018): 1055; F. Sassi et al., "Vitamin D: Nutrient, Hormone, and Immunomodulator," *Nutrients* 10, no. 11 (2018): 1656; Y. Hu et al., "Effect of Selenium on Thyroid Autoimmunity and Regulatory T Cells in Patients with Hashimoto's Thyroiditis: A Prospective Randomized-Controlled Trial," *Clinical and Translational Science* 14, no. 4 (2021): 1390–402; C. Mölzer et al., "A Role for Folate in Microbiome-Linked Control of Autoimmunity," *Journal of Immunology Research* 2021 (2021).

6. GG Konijeti et al., "Efficacy of the Autoimmune Protocol Diet for Inflammatory Bowel Disease," *Inflammatory Bowel Diseases* 23, no. 11 (2017): 2054–60; A. Chandrasekaran et al., "The Autoimmune Protocol Diet Modifies Intestinal RNA Expression in Inflammatory Bowel Disease," *Crohn's & Colitis 360* 1, no. 3 (2019): otz016; A. Chandrasekaran et al., "An Autoimmune Protocol Diet Improves Patient-Reported Quality of Life in Inflammatory Bowel Disease," *Crohn's & Colitis 360* 1, no. 3 (2019): otz019; RD Abbott et al., "Efficacy of the Autoimmune Protocol Diet as Part of a Multi-disciplinary, Supported Lifestyle Intervention for Hashimoto's Thyroiditis," *Cureus* 11, no. 4 (2019): e4556.

7. C. Catassi et al., "Coeliac Disease," *Lancet* 399, no. 10344 (2022): 2413–26.

8. C. Sategna-Guidetti et al., "Autoimmune Thyroid Diseases and Coeliac Disease," *European Journal of Gastroenterology & Hepatology* 10, no. 11 (1998): 927–31; E. Kowalska et al., "Estimation of Antithyroid Antibodies Occurrence in Children with Coeliac Disease," *Medical Science Monitor: International Medical Journal of Experimental and Clinical Research* 6, no. 4 (2000): 719–21; D. Larizza et al., "Celiac Disease in Children with Autoimmune Thyroid Disease," *Journal of Pediatrics* 139, no. 5 (2001): 738–40; M. Hakanen et al., "Clinical and

Subclinical Autoimmune Thyroid Disease in Adult Celiac Disease,"
Digestive Diseases and Sciences 46 (2001): 2631–35; MN Akçay, "The
Presence of the Antigliadin Antibodies in Autoimmune Thyroid
Diseases," *Hepatogastroenterology* 50, no. 2 (2003): cclxxix–cclxxx; TG
Strieder et al., "Risk Factors for and Prevalence of Thyroid Disorders in
a Cross-Sectional Study Among Healthy Female Relatives of Patients
with Autoimmune Thyroid Disease," *Clinical Endocrinology* 59, no. 3
(2003): 396–401; CL Ch'ng et al., "Prospective Screening for Coeliac
Disease in Patients with Graves' Hyperthyroidism Using Anti-gliadin
and Tissue Transglutaminase Antibodies," *Clinical Endocrinology* 62,
no. 3 (2005): 303–306; AJ Naiyer et al., "Tissue Transglutaminase
Antibodies in Individuals with Celiac Disease Bind to Thyroid Follicles
and Extracellular Matrix and May Contribute to Thyroid Dysfunction,"
Thyroid 18 (2008):1171–78; RK Marwaha et al., "Glutamic Acid
Decarboxylase (anti-GAD) & Tissue Transglutaminase (anti-TTG)
Antibodies in Patients with Thyroid Autoimmunity," *Indian Journal
of Medical Research* 137, no. 1 (2013): 82; I. Sange et al., "Celiac
Disease and the Autoimmune Web of Endocrinopathies," *Cureus* 12,
no. 12 (2020): e12383; M. Van der Pals et al., "Prevalence of Thyroid
Autoimmunity in Children with Celiac Disease Compared to Healthy
12-Year-Olds," *Autoimmune Diseases* 2014 (2014); A. Meloni et al.,
"Prevalence of Autoimmune Thyroiditis in Children with Celiac
Disease and Effect of Gluten Withdrawal," *Journal of Pediatrics* 155,
no. 1 (2009): 51–55; T. Ashok et al., "Celiac Disease and Autoimmune
Thyroid Disease: The Two Peas in a Pod," *Cureus* 14, no. 6 (2022):
e26243.

9. C. Sategna-Guidetti et al., "Autoimmune Thyroid Diseases and Coeliac
Disease," *European Journal of Gastroenterology & Hepatology* 10, no. 11
(1998): 927–31; RK Marwaha et al., "Glutamic Acid Decarboxylase
(anti-GAD) & Tissue Transglutaminase (anti-TTG) Antibodies in
Patients with Thyroid Autoimmunity," *Indian Journal of Medical
Research* 137, no. 1 (2013): 82; L. Salarian et al., "Extra-intestinal
Manifestations of Celiac Disease in Children: Their Prevalence and
Association with Human Leukocyte Antigens and Pathological and
Laboratory Evaluations," *BMC Pediatrics* 23, no. 1 (2023): 8.

10. A. Katz et al., "Celiac Disease Associated with Immune Complex
Glomerulonephritis," *Clinical Nephrology* 11, no. 1 (1979): 39–44.

11. L. Gamlin et al., "Food Sensitivity and Rheumatoid Arthritis,"
Environmental Toxicology and Pharmacology 4, no. 1–2 (1997): 43–49.

12. T. Watts et al., "Role of the Intestinal Tight Junction Modulator
Zonulin in the Pathogenesis of Type I Diabetes in BB Diabetic-Prone
Rats," *Proceedings of the National Academy of Sciences* 102, no. 8 (2005):

2916–21; S. Drago et al., "Gliadin, Zonulin and Gut Permeability: Effects on Celiac and Non-celiac Intestinal Mucosa and Intestinal Cell Lines," *Scandinavian Journal of Gastroenterology* 41, no. 4 (2006): 408–19; A. Sapone et al., "Zonulin Upregulation Is Associated with Increased Gut Permeability in Subjects with Type 1 Diabetes and Their Relatives," *Diabetes* 55, no. 5 (2006): 1443–49; MA Odenwald et al., "Intestinal Permeability Defects: Is It Time to Treat?" *Clinical Gastroenterology and Hepatology* 11, no. 9 (2013): 1075–83; K. Khoshbin et al., "Effects of Dietary Components on Intestinal Permeability in Health and Disease," *American Journal of Physiology-Gastrointestinal and Liver Physiology* 319, no. 5 (2020): G589–608.

13. A. Fasano, "All Disease Begins in the (Leaky) Gut: Role of Zonulin-Mediated Gut Permeability in the Pathogenesis of Some Chronic Inflammatory Diseases," *F1000Research* 9 (2020).

14. Key nutrients that can help with gut health and barrier integrity and may help in supplement form. L-glutamine is the amino acid with the most evidence. It gets consumed at higher rates when your body is stressed. L-glutamine is a key source of energy for the lining of the gut, including both enterocytes and immune cells. All amino acids should be consumed on an empty stomach.

   Vitamin A
   Vitamin D
   Curcumin (see chapter 10)
   Zinc
   Vitamin B9 (folate)
   Butyric acid
   Omega-3
   CLA
   Amino acids: L-glutamine, L-arginine, L-tryptophan, L-citruline
   Collagen peptides
   Triphala if constipated
   Deglycyrrhized licorice
   Berberine
   Prebiotics
   Probiotics

15. For more information on how to work with a functional medicine clinician, go to the Institute of Functional Medicine, IFM.org, and search "Find a Practitioner" for someone in your area.

16. Y. Ma et al., "Association Between Dietary Fiber and Markers of Systemic Inflammation in the Women's Health Initiative Observational Study," *Nutrition* 24 (2008): 941–49.

17. D. Furman et al., "Chronic Inflammation in the Etiology of Disease Across the Life Span," *Nature Medicine* 25, no. 12 (2019): 1822–32.

Chapter 9: Sleep and Stress Protocol

1. DB O'Connor et al., "Stress, Cortisol and Suicide Risk," *International Review of Neurobiology* 152 (2020): 101–30.

2. Ehlers-Danlos Syndrome (EDS) and Sjögren's syndrome. EDS is a group of genetic connective tissue disorders that include skin hyperelasticity, hypermobile joints, atrophic scarring, and fragile blood vessels. Some people consider EDS to have an autoimmune component. Sjögren's syndrome is an autoimmune disorder characterized by dry eyes and a dry mouth. It commonly occurs with other autoimmune conditions, such as rheumatoid arthritis and lupus.

3. PJ Colvonen et al., "Obstructive Sleep Apnea and Posttraumatic Stress Disorder Among OEF/OIF/OND Veterans," *Journal of Clinical Sleep Medicine* 11, no. 5 (2015): 513–18; P. Katz et al., "Sleep Disorders Among Individuals with Rheumatoid Arthritis," *Arthritis Care and Research* (2022).

4. YH Hsiao et al., "Sleep Disorders and Increased Risk of Autoimmune Diseases in Individuals Without Sleep Apnea," *Sleep* 38, no. 4 (2015): 581–86.

5. KA Babson et al., "Temporal Relations Between Sleep Problems and Both Traumatic Event Exposure and PTSD: A Critical Review of the Empirical Literature," *Journal of Anxiety Disorders* 24, no.1 (2010): 1–15; B. Kleim et al., "Effects of Sleep after Experimental Trauma on Intrusive Emotional Memories," *Sleep* 39, no. 12 (2016): 2125–32; T. Mollayeva et al., "Post-Traumatic Sleep-Wake Disorders," *Current Neurology and Neuroscience Reports* 17 (2017): 1–23.

6. DP Chapman et al., "Adverse Childhood Experiences and Sleep Disturbances in Adults," *Sleep Medicine* 12, no. 8 (2011): 773–79; RC Brindle et al., "The Relationship Between Childhood Trauma and Poor Sleep Health in Adulthood," *Psychosomatic Medicine* 80, no. 2 (2018): 200–207; K. Sullivan et al., "Adverse Childhood Experiences Affect Sleep Duration for Up to 50 Years Later," *Sleep* 42, no. 7 (2019): zsz087.

7. V. Mysliwiec et al., "Trauma Associated Sleep Disorder: A Parasomnia Induced by Trauma," *Sleep Medicine Reviews* 37 (2018): 94–104.

8. B. Kleim et al., "Effects of Sleep after Experimental Trauma on Intrusive Emotional Memories," *Sleep* 39, no. 12 (2016): 2125–32.

9. DJ Miller et al., "A Validation of Six Wearable Devices for Estimating Sleep, Heart Rate and Heart Rate Variability in Healthy Adults," *Sensors* 22, no. 16 (2022): 6317.

10. M. Altini et al., "The Promise of Sleep: A Multi-Sensor Approach for Accurate Sleep Stage Detection Using the Oura Ring," *Sensors* 22, no. 13 (2021): 4302; S. Ghorbani et al., "Multi-Night At-Home Evaluation of Improved Sleep Detection and Classification with a

Memory-Enhanced Consumer Sleep Tracker," *Nature and Science of Sleep* 14 (2022): 645.

11. ML Sambou et al., "Investigation of the Relationships Between Sleep Behaviors and Risk of Healthspan Termination: A Prospective Cohort Study Based on 323,373 UK-Biobank Participants," *Sleep Breath* 26, no. 1 (2022): 205–13.

12. State of New Hampshire Employee Assistance Program, "Perceived Stress Scale," https://www.das.nh.gov/wellness/Docs%5CPercieved%20Stress%20Scale.pdf. Or try the one hosted by Mind Garden: S. Cohen, "Perceived Stress Scale," https://www.mindgarden.com/documents/PerceivedStressScale.pdf.

13. HG Kim et al., "Stress and Heart Rate Variability: A Meta-Analysis and Review of the Literature," *Psychiatry Investigation* 15, no. 3 (2018): 235.

14. "Female Hormone Optimization," Huberman Lab, January 30, 2023, https://hubermanlab.com/dr-sara-gottfried-how-to-optimize-female-hormone-health-for-vitality-and-longevity/.

15. MY Balban et al., "Brief Structured Respiration Practices Enhance Mood and Reduce Physiological Arousal," *Cell Reports Medicine* (2023): 100895.

Chapter 10: Immunomodulator Protocol

1. A. Samsel et al., "Glyphosate, Pathways to Modern Diseases II: Celiac Sprue and Gluten Intolerance," *Interdisciplinary Toxicology* 6, no. 4 (2013): 159–84; L. Zhang et al., "Exposure to Glyphosate-Based Herbicides and Risk for Non-Hodgkin Lymphoma: A Meta-Analysis and Supporting Evidence," *Mutation Research/Reviews in Mutation Research* 781 (2019): 186–206; M. Pahwa et al., "Glyphosate Use and Associations with Non-Hodgkin Lymphoma Major Histological Sub-Types: Findings from the North American Pooled Project," *Scandinavian Journal of Work, Environment & Health* 45, no. 6 (2019): 600–609; DD Weisenburger, "A Review and Update with Perspective of Evidence that the Herbicide Glyphosate (Roundup) Is a Cause of Non-Hodgkin Lymphoma," *Clinical Lymphoma Myeloma and Leukemia* 21, no. 9 (2021): 621–30; GC Kabat et al., "On Recent Meta-Analyses of Exposure to Glyphosate and Risk of Non-Hodgkin's Lymphoma in Humans," *Cancer Causes & Control* 32 (2021): 409–14; F. Meloni et al., "Occupational Exposure to Glyphosate and Risk of Lymphoma: Results of an Italian Multicenter Case-Control Study," *Environmental Health* 20, no. 1 (2021): 1–8.

2. R. Mesnage et al., "Impacts of Dietary Exposure to Pesticides on Faecal Microbiome Metabolism in Adult Twins," *Environmental Health* 21, no. 1 (2022): 1–14.

3. "Overall, our review did not find support in the epidemiologic literature
    for a causal association between glyphosate and non-Hodgkin's
    lymphoma or multiple myeloma." J. Acquavella et al., "Glyphosate
    Epidemiology Expert Panel Review: A Weight of Evidence Systematic
    Review of the Relationship Between Glyphosate Exposure and Non-
    Hodgkin's Lymphoma or Multiple Myeloma," *Critical Reviews in
    Toxicology* 46, supp. 1(2016): 28–43.

    "In this large, prospective cohort study, no association was apparent
    between glyphosate and any solid tumors or lymphoid malignancies
    overall, including NHL and its subtypes. There was some evidence of
    increased risk of AML among the highest exposed group that requires
    confirmation." G. Andreotti et al., "Glyphosate Use and Cancer
    Incidence in the Agricultural Health Study," *JNCI: Journal of the
    National Cancer Institute* 110, no. 5 (2018): 509–16.

    "Our meta-analysis provided no overall evidence of an increased
    risk for both NHL and MM in subjects occupationally exposed to
    glyphosate. In secondary analyses we detected a small increase in risk
    for the category with highest level of exposure as well as for diffuse large
    B-cell lymphoma (DLBCL)." F. Donato et al., "Exposure to Glyphosate
    and Risk of Non-Hodgkin Lymphoma and Multiple Myeloma: An
    Updated Meta-Analysis," *La Medicina del Lavoro* 111, no. 1 (2020): 63.

    "This updated meta-analysis reinforces our previous conclusion of a
    lack of an association between exposure to glyphosate and risk of NHL
    overall, although an association with DLBCL cannot be ruled out."
    P. Boffetta et al., "Exposure to Glyphosate and Risk of Non-Hodgkin
    Lymphoma: An Updated Meta-Analysis," *La Medicina del Lavoro* 112,
    no. 3 (2021): 194.

4. P. López et al., "Intestinal Dysbiosis in Systemic Lupus Erythematosus:
    Cause or Consequence?," *Current Opinion in Rheumatology* 28,
    no. 5 (2016): 515–22; KC Navegantes et al., "Immune Modulation
    of Some Autoimmune Diseases: The Critical Role of Macrophages
    and Neutrophils in the Innate and Adaptive Immunity," *Journal of
    Translational Medicine* 15, no. 1 (2017): 1–21; F. De Luca et al.,
    "The Microbiome in Autoimmune Diseases," *Clinical & Experimental
    Immunology* 195, no. 1 (2019): 74–85.

5. Toll-like receptors (TLRs) play a key role in stimulation of the innate
    immune response and inflammation. TLRs can be categorized as (1)
    extracellular TLRs that recognize microbial membrane components
    (TLR1, 2, 4, 5, 6, and 10), and (2) intracellular TLRs that recognize
    microbial nucleic acids (TLR3, 7, 8, and 9). Curcumin is a dietary
    polyphenol from *Curcuma longa L.* that offers myriad biological
    effects. Research demonstrates that polyphenols like curcumin have a

dampening effect on the toll-like receptor (TLR) signaling pathways, specifically in TLR-2 and TLR-4 activation, suggesting its role in reducing overall inflammatory burden, particularly for autoimmune and rheumatic diseases.

AM Krieg et al., "Toll-Like Receptors 7, 8, and 9: Linking Innate Immunity to Autoimmunity," *Immunological Reviews* 220, no. 1 (2007): 251–69; CY Chen et al., "The Cancer Prevention, Anti-Inflammatory and Anti-Oxidation of Bioactive Phytochemicals Targeting the TLR4 Signaling Pathway," *International Journal of Molecular Sciences* 19, no. 9 (2018): 2729; MA Panaro et al., "The Emerging Role of Curcumin in the Modulation of TLR-4 Signaling Pathway: Focus on Neuroprotective and Anti-Rheumatic Properties," *International Journal of Molecular Sciences* 21, no. 7 (2020): 2299; A. Ebrahimzadeh et al., "Effects of Curcumin Supplementation on Inflammatory Biomarkers in Patients with Rheumatoid Arthritis and Ulcerative Colitis: A Systematic Review and Meta-Analysis," *Complementary Therapies in Medicine* 61 (2021): 102773; KS Coutinho-Wolino et al., "Bioactive Compounds Modulating Toll-Like 4 Receptor (TLR4)-Mediated Inflammation: Pathways Involved and Future Perspectives," *Nutrition Research* (2022); D. Beghelli et al., "Dietary Supplementation with Boswellia Serrata, Verbascum Thapsus, and Curcuma Longa in Show Jumping Horses: Effects on Serum Proteome, Antioxidant Status, and Anti-Inflammatory Gene Expression," *Life* 13, no. 3 (2023): 750.

6. SL Galetta, "The Controlled High Risk Avonex Multiple Sclerosis Trial (CHAMPS Study)," *Journal of Neuro-Ophthalmology* 21, no. 4 (2001): 292–95; MC Genovese et al., "A Randomized, Controlled Trial of Interferon-beta-1a (Avonex(R)) in Patients with Rheumatoid Arthritis: A Pilot Study [ISRCTN03626626]," *Arthritis Research Therapies* 6, no. 1 (2003): 1–5; RM Herndon et al., "Eight-Year Immunogenicity and Safety of Interferon beta-1a-Avonex Treatment in Patients with Multiple Sclerosis," *Multiple Sclerosis Journal* 11, no. 4 (2005): 409–19; G. Comi et al., "Safety and Efficacy of Ozanimod Versus Interferon beta-1a in Relapsing Multiple Sclerosis (SUNBEAM): A Multicentre, Randomised, Minimum 12-month, Phase 3 Trial," *Lancet Neurology* 18, no. 11 (2019): 1009–20; SL Cohan et al., "Interferons and Multiple Sclerosis: Lessons from 25 Years of Clinical and Real-World Experience with Intramuscular Interferon Beta-1a (Avonex)," *CNS Drugs* 35, no. 7 (2021): 743–67.

7. N. Shivappa et al., "Designing and Developing a Literature-Derived, Population-Based Dietary Inflammatory Index," *Public Health Nutrition* 17, no. 8 (2014): 1689–96; M. Gabriele et al., "Diet Bioactive Compounds: Implications for Oxidative Stress and Inflammation in

the Vascular System," *Endocrine, Metabolic & Immune Disorders—Drug Targets* 17, no. 4 (2017): 264–75; D. Furman et al., "Chronic Inflammation in the Etiology of Disease Across the Life Span," *Nature Medicine* 25, no. 12 (2019): 1822–32.

8. D. Odobasic et al., "Neutrophil-Mediated Regulation of Innate and Adaptive Immunity: The Role of Myeloperoxidase," *Journal of Immunology Research* 2016 (2016).

9. F.O. Buendía-González et al., "The Similarities and Differences Between the Effects of Testosterone and DHEA on the Innate and Adaptive Immune Response," *Biomolecules* 12, no. 12 (2022): 1768.

10. I recommend going to survivingmold.com and taking their visual contrast sensitivity (VCS) test. It costs $15. https://www.survivingmold.com/store/online-vcs-screening.

11. SG Wannamethee et al., "Associations of Vitamin C Status, Fruit and Vegetable Intakes, and Markers of Inflammation and Hemostasis," *American Journal of Clinical Nutrition* 83, no. 3 (2006): 567–74; E. Mah et al., "Vitamin C Status Is Related to Proinflammatory Responses and Impaired Vascular Endothelial Function in Healthy, College-Aged Lean and Obese Men," *Journal of the American Dietetic Association* 111, no. 5 (2011): 737–43; AW Ashor et al., "Effect of Vitamin C and Vitamin E Supplementation on Endothelial Function: A Systematic Review and Meta-Analysis of Randomised Controlled Trials," *British Journal of Nutrition* 113, no. 8 (2015): 1182–94.

12. AW Ashor et al., "Effect of Vitamin C and Vitamin E Supplementation on Endothelial Function: A Systematic Review and Meta-Analysis of Randomised Controlled Trials," *British Journal of Nutrition* 113, no. 8 (2015): 1182–94.

13. PC Calder, "Omega-3 Fatty Acids and Inflammatory Processes," *Nutrients* 2, no. 3 (2010): 355–74.

14. Read more about vitamins A and D and their role in the gut and immune system in these recent reviews: R. Farré et al., "Intestinal Permeability, Inflammation and the Role of Nutrients," *Nutrients* 12, no. 4 (2020): 1185; K. Khoshbin et al., "Effects of Dietary Components on Intestinal Permeability in Health and Disease," *American Journal of Physiology-Gastrointestinal and Liver Physiology* 319, no. 5 (2020): G589–G608.

15. K. Osowiecka et al., "The Influence of Nutritional Intervention in the Treatment of Hashimoto's Thyroiditis—A Systematic Review," *Nutrients* 15, no. 4 (2023): 1041.

16. MA Farhangi et al., "The Effects of Nigella Sativa on Thyroid Function, Serum Vascular Endothelial Growth Factor (VEGF)–1, Nesfatin-1 and Anthropometric Features in Patients with Hashimoto's Thyroiditis: A

Randomized Controlled Trial," *BMC Complementary and Alternative Medicine* 16 (2016): 1–9; MA Farhangi et al., "The Effects of Powdered Black Cumin Seeds on Markers of Oxidative Stress, Intracellular Adhesion Molecule (ICAM)-1 and Vascular Cell Adhesion Molecule (VCAM)-1 in Patients with Hashimoto's Thyroiditis," *Clinical Nutrition ESPEN* 37 (2020): 207–12; MA Farhangi et al., "Powdered Black Cumin Seeds Strongly Improves Serum Lipids, Atherogenic Index of Plasma and Modulates Anthropometric Features in Patients with Hashimoto's Thyroiditis," *Lipids in Health and Disease* 17 (2018): 1–7.

17. MA Farhangi et al., "Powdered Black Cumin Seeds Strongly Improves Serum Lipids, Atherogenic Index of Plasma and Modulates Anthropometric Features in Patients with Hashimoto's Thyroiditis," *Lipids in Health and Disease* 17 (2018): 1–7.

18. M. Zielińska et al., "The Role of Bioactive Compounds of *Nigella sativa* in Rheumatoid Arthritis Therapy-Current Reports," *Nutrients* 13, no. 10 (2021): 3369.

19. AF Majdalawieh et al., "Immunomodulatory and Anti-inflammatory Action of Nigella sativa and Thymoquinone: A Comprehensive Review," *International Immunopharmacology* 28, no. 1 (2015): 295–304.

20. The four categories of polyphenols are flavonoids (includes quercetin, catechins, anthocyanins, found in leafy vegetables, berries, citrus, apples, onion, tea, dark chocolate, and red cabbage), phenolic acid (includes stilbenes and lignans found in the skins of fruits and leaves of vegetables, and seeds like flax and sesame), polyphenolic amides (includes capsaicinoids found in chili peppers as an example), and other (resveratrol in red wine, and curcumin in turmeric).
AN Panche et al., "Flavonoids: An Overview," *Journal of Nutritional Science* 5 (2016): e47; B. Kocaadam et al., "Curcumin, An Active Component of Turmeric (Curcuma longa), and Its Effects on Health," *Critical Reviews in Food Science and Nutrition* 57, no. 13 (2017): 2889–95; C. Di Lorenzo et al., "Polyphenols and Human Health: The Role of Bioavailability," *Nutrients* 13, no. 1 (2021): 273.

21. Y. Kim et al., "Polyphenols and Glycemic Control," *Nutrients* 8, no. 1 (2016): 17; M. Shahwan et al., "Role of Polyphenols in Combating Type 2 Diabetes and Insulin Resistance," *International Journal of Biological Macromolecules* (2022); S. Wang et al., "Natural Polyphenols: A Potential Prevention and Treatment Strategy for Metabolic Syndrome," *Food & Function* 13, no. 19 (2022): 9734–53.

22. DJ Jiang et al., "Pharmacological Effects of Xanthones as Cardiovascular Protective Agents," *Cardiovascular Drug Reviews* 22, no. 2 (2004): 91–102; ML Garg et al., "Macadamia Nut Consumption Modulates Favourably Risk Factors for Coronary Artery Disease in

Hypercholesterolemic Subjects," *Lipids* 42, no. 6 (2007): 583–87; AB Santhakumar et al., "A Review of the Mechanisms and Effectiveness of Dietary Polyphenols in Reducing Oxidative Stress and Thrombotic Risk," *Journal of Human Nutrition and Dietetics* 27, no. 1 (2014): 1–21; F. Tamer et al., "Nutrition Phytochemicals Affecting Platelet Signaling and Responsiveness: Implications for Thrombosis and Hemostasis," *Thrombosis and Haemostasis* (2021).

23. C. Sandoval-Acuña et al., "Polyphenols and Mitochondria: An Update on Their Increasingly Emerging ROS-Scavenging Independent Actions," *Archives of Biochemistry and Biophysics* 559 (2014): 75–90; FR Jardim et al., "Resveratrol and Brain Mitochondria: A Review," *Molecular Neurobiology* 55 (2018): 2085–101; J. Teixeira et al., "Dietary Polyphenols and Mitochondrial Function: Role in Health and Disease," *Current Medicinal Chemistry* 26, no. 19 (2019): 3376–406; M. Naoi et al:, "Mitochondria in Neuroprotection by Phytochemicals: Bioactive Polyphenols Modulate Mitochondrial Apoptosis System, Function and Structure," *International Journal of Molecular Sciences* 20, no. 10 (2019): 2451; H. Bhagani et al., "The Mitochondria: A Target of Polyphenols in the Treatment of Diabetic Cardiomyopathy," *International Journal of Molecular Sciences* 21, no. 14 (2020): 4962; F. Ashkar et al., "The Effect of Polyphenols on Kidney Disease: Targeting Mitochondria," *Nutrients* 14, no. 15 (2022): 3115.

24. SK Nicholson et al., "Effects of Dietary Polyphenols on Gene Expression in Human Vascular Endothelial Cells," *Proceedings of the Nutrition Society* 67, no. 1 (2008): 42–47; J. Joven et al; "Bioactive Food Components Platform. Polyphenols and the Modulation of Gene Expression Pathways: Can We Eat Our Way out of the Danger of Chronic Disease?," *Critical Reviews in Food Science and Nutrition* 54, no. 8 (2014): 985–1001; G. Qu et al., "The Beneficial and Deleterious Role of Dietary Polyphenols on Chronic Degenerative Diseases by Regulating Gene Expression," *Bioscience Trends* 12, no. 6 (2018): 526–36; GG Kang et al., "Dietary Polyphenols and Gene Expression in Molecular Pathways Associated with Type 2 Diabetes Mellitus: A Review," *International Journal of Molecular Sciences* 21, no. 1 (2019): 140; E. Cione et al., "Quercetin, Epigallocatechin Gallate, Curcumin, and Resveratrol: From Dietary Sources to Human MicroRNA Modulation," *Molecules* 25, no. 1 (2019): 63; A. Nani et al., "Antioxidant and Anti-Inflammatory Potential of Polyphenols Contained in Mediterranean Diet in Obesity: Molecular Mechanisms," *Molecules* 26, no. 4 (2021): 985; T. Bhattacharya et al., "Role of Phytonutrients in Nutrigenetics and Nutrigenomics Perspective in Curing Breast Cancer," *Biomolecules* 11, no. 8 (2021): 1176.

25. A. Nani et al., "Antioxidant and Anti-Inflammatory Potential of Polyphenols Contained in Mediterranean Diet in Obesity: Molecular Mechanisms," *Molecules* 26, no. 4 (2021): 985; D. Cianciosi et al., "The Reciprocal Interaction Between Polyphenols and Other Dietary Compounds: Impact on Bioavailability, Antioxidant Capacity and Other Physico-chemical and Nutritional Parameters," *Food Chemistry* 375 (2022): 131904; A. Rana et al., "Health Benefits of Polyphenols: A Concise Review," *Journal of Food Biochemistry* 46, no. 10 (2022): e14264.

26. JJ Bright, "Curcumin and Autoimmune Disease," *Advances in Experimental Medicine and Biology* 595 (2007): 425–51; GT Diaz-Gerevini et al., "Beneficial Action of Resveratrol: How and Why?," *Nutrition* 32, no. 2 (2016): 174–78; H. Khan et al., "Polyphenols in the Treatment of Autoimmune Diseases," *Autoimmunity Reviews* 18, no. 7 (2019): 647–57; S. Wang et al., "Immunomodulatory Effects of Green Tea Polyphenols," *Molecules* 26, no. 12 (2021): 3755; H. Shakoor et al., "Immunomodulatory Effects of Dietary Polyphenols," *Nutrients* 13, no. 3 (2021): 728.

27. I recommend this recipe for kitchari to my autoimmune patients and eat it a lot myself!

    2 tablespoons ghee

    Turmeric root, peeled and chopped to taste (I use about 2 tablespoons)

    2 teaspoons each of black mustard seeds, cumin seeds, and black pepper

    2 bay leaves

    1 teaspoon each of coriander powder, cumin powder, fennel seeds, and fenugreek seeds

    2 cups mung dal beans, rinsed until water runs clear

    6 to 8 cups filtered water or bone broth

    4 to 6 cups chopped seasonal vegetables, such as burdock root, greens, carrots, squash (avoid nightshades, such as tomatoes, potatoes, and chiles)

    1 cup fresh cilantro, chopped

    Heat the ghee in a large pot. Add the seeds and cook until mustard seeds pop in delight. Add bay leaves and powdered spices. Add mung dal, then the water or broth. Bring to a boil, then lower to simmer. Cook to desired doneness of beans—I typically cook for 30 minutes to porridge consistency, then add vegetables. I like for vegetables to be a bit crispy, so I cook for another 10 to 15 minutes only. Serve with cilantro as a garnish.

28. Curcumin lowers inflammation as measured by CRP and ESR in

patients with rheumatoid arthritis and ulcerative colitis.
A. Ebrahimzadeh et al., "Effects of Curcumin Supplementation on Inflammatory Biomarkers in Patients with Rheumatoid Arthritis and Ulcerative Colitis: A Systematic Review and Meta-Analysis," *Complementary Therapies in Medicine* 61 (2021): 102773.

29. MC Szymanski et al., "Short-Term Dietary Curcumin Supplementation Reduces Gastrointestinal Barrier Damage and Physiological Strain Responses During Exertional Heat Stress," *Journal of Applied Physiology* 124, no. 2 (2018): 330–40.

30. SY Lee et al., "Epigallocatechin-3-Gallate Ameliorates Autoimmune Arthritis by Reciprocal Regulation of T Helper-17 Regulatory T Cells and Inhibition of Osteoclastogenesis by Inhibiting STAT3 Signaling," *Journal of Leucocyte Biology* 100, no. 3 (2016): 559–68; M. Aparicio-Soto et al., "An Update on Diet and Nutritional Factors in Systemic Lupus Erythematosus Management," *Nutrition Research Reviews* 30, no. 1 (2017): 118–37; S. Wang et al., "Immunomodulatory Effects of Green Tea Polyphenols," *Molecules* 26, no. 12 (2021): 3755; F. Cai et al., "Epigallocatechin-3 Gallate Regulates Macrophage Subtypes and Immunometabolism to Ameliorate Experimental Autoimmune Encephalomyelitis," *Cellular Immunology* 368 (2021): 104421; T. Behl et al., "Exploring the Role of Polyphenols in Rheumatoid Arthritis," *Critical Reviews in Food Science and Nutrition* 62, no. 19 (2022): 5372–93.

31. Y. Li et al., "Quercetin, Inflammation and Immunity," *Nutrients* 8, no. 3 (2016): 167; YL Lyu et al., "Biological Activities Underlying the Therapeutic Effect of Quercetin on Inflammatory Bowel Disease," *Mediators of Inflammation* 2022 (2022); K. Yuan et al., "Quercetin Alleviates Rheumatoid Arthritis by Inhibiting Neutrophil Inflammatory Activities," *Journal of Nutritional Biochemistry* 84 (2020): 108454; HT Sun et al., "Quercetin Suppresses Inflammatory Cytokine Production in Rheumatoid Arthritis Fibroblast-Like Synoviocytes," *Experimental and Therapeutic Medicine* 22, no. 5 (2021): 1–7; P. Shen et al., "Potential Implications of Quercetin in Autoimmune Diseases," *Frontiers in Immunology* (2021): 1991; F. Guan et al., "Anti-Rheumatic Effect of Quercetin and Recent Developments in Nano Formulation," *RSC Advances* 11, no. 13 (2021): 7280–93.

32. JL Bitterman et al., "Metabolic Effects of Resveratrol: Addressing the Controversies," *Cellular and Molecular Life Sciences* 72 (2015): 1473–88; GP Dias et al., "Resveratrol: A Potential Hippocampal Plasticity Enhancer," *Oxidative Medicine and Cellular Longevity* 2016 (2016); S. Weiskirchen et al., "Resveratrol: How Much Wine Do You Have to Drink to Stay Healthy?," *Advances in Nutrition* 7, no. 4 (2016):

706–18; SH Lee et al., "Sirtuin Signaling in Cellular Senescence and Aging," *BMB Reports* 52, no. 1 (2019): 24; JM Pezzuto, "Resveratrol: Twenty Years of Growth, Development and Controversy," *Biomolecules & Therapeutics* 27, no. 1 (2019): 1; A. Shaito et al., "Potential Adverse Effects of Resveratrol: A Literature Review," *International Journal of Molecular Sciences* 21, no. 6 (2020): 2084.

33. ALB Oliveira et al., "Resveratrol Role in Autoimmune Disease—A Mini-Review," *Nutrients* 9, no. 12 (2017): 1306; L. Malaguarnera, "Influence of Resveratrol on the Immune Response," *Nutrients* 11, no. 5 (2019): 946; S. Sheng et al., "The Role of Resveratrol on Rheumatoid Arthritis: From Bench to Bedside," *Frontiers in Pharmacology* 13 (2022).

34. ALB Oliveira et al., "Resveratrol Role in Autoimmune Disease—A Mini-Review," *Nutrients* 9, no. 12 (2017): 1306; Institute for Functional Medicine, "The Functional Medicine Approach to COVID-19: Additional Research on Nutraceuticals and Botanicals," https://www.ifm.org/news-insights/functional-medicine-approach-covid-19-additional-research-nutraceuticals-botanicals/.

35. MA Kriegel et al., "Does Vitamin D Affect Risk of Developing Autoimmune Disease?: A Systematic Review," *Seminars in Arthritis and Rheumatism* 40, no. 6 (2011): 512–31.

36. Ibid.; J. Hahn et al., "Vitamin D and Marine Omega 3 Fatty Acid Supplementation and Incident Autoimmune Disease: VITAL Randomized Controlled Trial," *BMJ* 376 (2022).

37. J. Hahn et al., "Vitamin D and Marine Omega 3 Fatty Acid Supplementation and Incident Autoimmune Disease: VITAL Randomized Controlled Trial," *BMJ* 376 (2022).

38. "Observational studies have found conflicting results; small trials of vitamin D supplementation in people with established autoimmune disease have mainly reported disappointing results." Ibid. Here is a selection: KH Costenbader et al., "Geographic Variation in Rheumatoid Arthritis Incidence Among Women in the United States," *Archives of Internal Medicine* 168, no. 15 (2008): 1664–70; B. Altieri et al., "Does Vitamin D Play a Role in Autoimmune Endocrine Disorders? A Proof of Concept," *Reviews in Endocrine and Metabolic Disorders* 18 (2017): 335–46; R. Scragg, "Limitations of Vitamin D Supplementation Trials: Why Observational Studies Will Continue to Help Determine the Role of Vitamin D in Health," *Journal of Steroid Biochemistry and Molecular Biology* 177 (2018): 6–9; G. Murdaca et al., "Emerging Role of Vitamin D in Autoimmune Diseases: An Update on Evidence and Therapeutic Implications," *Autoimmunity Reviews* 18, no. 9 (2019): 102350; A. Giustina et al., "Consensus Statement from 2nd International Conference on Controversies in Vitamin D," *Reviews in Endocrine and*

Metabolic Disorders 21 (2020): 89–116; T. Skaaby et al., "Prospective Population-Based Study of the Association Between Vitamin D Status and Incidence of Autoimmune Disease," *Endocrine* 50 (2015): 231–38.

39. "Vitamin D in particular may perturb viral cellular infection via interacting with cell entry receptors (angiotensin converting enzyme 2), ACE2." M. Iddir et al., "Strengthening the Immune System and Reducing Inflammation and Oxidative Stress Through Diet and Nutrition: Considerations During the COVID-19 Crisis," *Nutrients* 12, no. 6 (2020): 1562.

40. H. Kühne et al., "Vitamin D Receptor Knockout Mice Exhibit Elongated Intestinal Microvilli and Increased Ezrin Expression," *Nutrition Research* 36, no. 2 (2016): 184–92.

41. H. Zhao et al., "Protective Role of 1,25(OH)2 Vitamin D_3 in the Mucosal Injury and Epithelial Barrier Disruption in DSS-Induced Acute Colitis in Mice," *BMC Gastroenterology* 12, no. 1 (2012): 1–14.

42. H. Vargas-Robles et al., "Beneficial Effects of Nutritional Supplements on Intestinal Epithelial Barrier Functions in Experimental Colitis Models *in Vivo*," *World Journal of Gastroenterology* 25, no. 30 (2019): 4181.

43. "Short-term treatment with 2,000 international units (IU)/day of vitamin D or placebo for 3 months in patients with Crohn's disease has shown that vitamin D may improve gastroduodenal permeability (sucrose excretion) relative to the deterioration observed on placebo; however, there was no significant improvement in small intestinal or colonic permeability with vitamin D treatment for 3 months." T. Raftery et al., "Effects of Vitamin D Supplementation on Intestinal Permeability, Cathelicidin and Disease Markers in Crohn's Disease: Results from a Randomised Double-Blind Placebo-Controlled Study," *United European Gastroenterology Journal* 3, no. 3 (2015): 294–302.

44. W. Liu et al., "The Immunomodulatory Effect of Alpha-Lipoic Acid in Autoimmune Diseases," *BioMed Research International* 2019 (2019); M. Iddir et al., "Strengthening the Immune System and Reducing Inflammation and Oxidative Stress Through Diet and Nutrition: Considerations During the COVID-19 Crisis," *Nutrients* 12, no. 6 (2020): 1562; Z. Xie et al., "ROS-Dependent Lipid Peroxidation and Reliant Antioxidant Ferroptosis-Suppressor-Protein 1 in Rheumatoid Arthritis: A Covert Clue for Potential Therapy," *Inflammation* 44, no. 1 (2021): 35–47; D. Sharma et al., "Role of Natural Products in Alleviation of Rheumatoid Arthritis—A Review," *Journal of Food Biochemistry* 45, no. 4 (2021): e13673; Z. Xie et al., "Role of Lipoic Acid in Multiple Sclerosis," *CNS Neuroscience & Therapeutics* 28, no. 3 (2022): 319–31.

45. AA Shah et al., "Oxidative Stress and Autoimmune Skin Disease," *European Journal of Dermatology* 23, no. 1 (2013): 5–13; Y. Wang et al., "Perspectives of New Advances in the Pathogenesis of Vitiligo: From Oxidative Stress to Autoimmunity," *Medical Science Monitor: International Medical Journal of Experimental and Clinical Research* 25 (2019): 1017; Y. Zamudio-Cuevas et al., "Rheumatoid Arthritis and Oxidative Stress," *Cellular and Molecular Biology* 68, no. 6 (2022): 174–84.

46. Y. Wang et al., "Perspectives of New Advances in the Pathogenesis of Vitiligo: From Oxidative Stress to Autoimmunity," *Medical Science Monitor: International Medical Journal of Experimental and Clinical Research* 25 (2019): 1017; D. Li et al., "Vitiligo and Hashimoto's Thyroiditis: Autoimmune Diseases Linked by Clinical Presentation, Biochemical Commonality, and Autoimmune/Oxidative Stress-mediated Toxicity Pathogenesis," *Medical Hypotheses* 128 (2019): 69–75; S. Jarmakiewicz-Czaja et al., "Antioxidants as Protection against Reactive Oxidative Stress in Inflammatory Bowel Disease," *Metabolites* 13, no. 4 (2023): 573.

47. F. Cavalcoli et al., "Micronutrient Deficiencies in Patients with Chronic Atrophic Autoimmune Gastritis: A Review," *World Journal of Gastroenterology* 23, no. 4 (2017): 563–72.

48. K. Esalatmanesh et al., "Effects of N-acetylcysteine Supplementation on Disease Activity, Oxidative Stress, and Inflammatory and Metabolic Parameters in Rheumatoid Arthritis Patients: A Randomized Double-Blind Placebo-Controlled Trial," *Amino Acids* 54, no. 3 (2022): 433–40.

49. I prefer wild-caught salmon or other SMASH fish that are low in mercury: salmon, mackerel, anchovies, sardines, and herring.

50. JM Kremer et al., "Effects of Manipulation of Dietary Fatty Acids on Clinical Manifestations of Rheumatoid Arthritis," *The Lancet* 325, no. 8422 (1985): 184–87; JM Kremer et al., "Dietary Fish Oil and Olive Oil Supplementation in Patients with Rheumatoid Arthritis Clinical and Immunologic Effects," *Arthritis & Rheumatism: Official Journal of the American College of Rheumatology* 33, no. 6 (1990): 810–20; I. Nordvik et al., "Effect of Dietary Advice and N-3 Supplementation in Newly Diagnosed MS Patients," *Acta Neurologica Scandinavica* 102, no. 3 (2000): 143–49; E. Kouchaki et al., "High-Dose Omega-3 Fatty Acid Plus Vitamin D3 Supplementation Affects Clinical Symptoms and Metabolic Status of Patients with Multiple Sclerosis: A Randomized Controlled Clinical Trial," *Journal of Nutrition* 148, no. 8 (2018): 1380–86; S. Hoare et al., "Higher Intake of Omega-3 Polyunsaturated Fatty Acids Is Associated with a Decreased Risk of a First Clinical Diagnosis of Central Nervous System

Demyelination: Results from the Ausimmune Study," *Multiple Sclerosis Journal* 22, no. 7 (2016): 884–92; B. Weinstock-Guttman et al., "Low Fat Dietary Intervention with Omega-3 Fatty Acid Supplementation in Multiple Sclerosis Patients," *Prostaglandins, Leukotrienes and Essential Fatty Acids* 73, no. 5 (2005): 397–404; WF Clark et al., "Omega-3 Fatty Acid Dietary Supplementation in Systemic Lupus Erythematosus," *Kidney International* 36, no. 4 (1989): 653–60; G. Westberg et al., "Effect of MaxEPA in Patients with SLE. A Double-Blind, Crossover Study," *Scandinavian Journal of Rheumatology* 19, no. 2 (1990): 137–43; UN Das, "Beneficial Effect of Eicosapentaenoic and Docosahexaenoic Acids in the Management of Systemic Lupus Erythematosus and Its Relationship to the Cytokine Network," *Prostaglandins, Leukotrienes and Essential Fatty Acids* 51, no. 3 (1994): 207–13; EM Duffy et al., "The Clinical Effect of Dietary Supplementation with Omega-3 Fish Oils and/or Copper in Systemic Lupus Erythematosus," *Journal of Rheumatology* 31, no. 8 (2004): 1551–56; AC Elkan et al., "Diet and Fatty Acid Pattern Among Patients with SLE: Associations with Disease Activity, Blood Lipids and Atherosclerosis," *Lupus* 21, no. 13 (2012): 1405–11; C. Arriens et al., "Placebo-Controlled Randomized Clinical Trial of Fish Oil's Impact on Fatigue, Quality of Life, and Disease Activity in Systemic Lupus Erythematosus," *Nutrition Journal* 14 (2015): 1–11; KJ Bello et al., "Omega-3 in SLE: A Double-Blind, Placebo-Controlled Randomized Clinical Trial of Endothelial Dysfunction and Disease Activity in Systemic Lupus Erythematosus," *Rheumatology International* 33 (2013): 2789–96; O. Torkildsen et al., "Omega-3 Fatty Acid Treatment in Multiple Sclerosis (OFAMS Study) A Randomized, Double-Blind, Placebo-Controlled Trial," *Archives of Neurology* 69, no. 8 (2012): 1044–51; M. Veselinovic et al., "Clinical Benefits of N-3 PUFA and γ-Linolenic Acid in Patients with Rheumatoid Arthritis," *Nutrients* 9, no. 4 (2017): 325; WF Clark et al., "Omega-3 Fatty Acid Dietary Supplementation in Systemic Lupus Erythematosus," *Kidney International* 36, no. 4 (1989): 653–60; H. van der Tempel et al., "Effects of Fish Oil Supplementation in Rheumatoid Arthritis," *Annals of the Rheumatic Diseases* 49, no. 2 (1990): 76–80; L.C. Stene et al., "Use of Cod Liver Oil During the First Year of Life Is Associated with Lower Risk of Childhood-Onset Type 1 Diabetes: A Large, Population-Based, Case-Control Study," *American Journal of Clinical Nutrition* 78, no. 6 (2003): 1128–34; JM Norris et al., "Omega-3 Polyunsaturated Fatty Acid Intake and Islet Autoimmunity in Children at Increased Risk for Type 1 Diabetes," *JAMA* 298, no. 12 (2007): 1420–28; F. Cadario et al., "Administration of Vitamin D and High Dose of Omega 3 to Sustain Remission of Type

1 Diabetes," *European Review for Medical and Pharmacological Sciences* 22, no. 2 (2018): 512–15; HP Chase et al., "Effect of Docosahexaenoic Acid Supplementation on Inflammatory Cytokine Levels in Infants at High Genetic Risk for Type 1 Diabetes," *Pediatric Diabetes* 16, no. 4 (2015): 271–79; GT Espersen et al., "Decreased Interleukin-1 Beta Levels in Plasma from Rheumatoid Arthritis Patients After Dietary Supplementation with N-3 Polyunsaturated Fatty Acids," *Clinical Rheumatology* 11 (1992): 393–95; YH Lee et al., "Omega-3 Polyunsaturated Fatty Acids and the Treatment of Rheumatoid Arthritis: A Meta-Analysis," *Archives of Medical Research* 43, no. 5 (2012): 356–62; U. Akbar et al., "Omega-3 Fatty Acids in Rheumatic Diseases: A Critical Review," *JCR: Journal of Clinical Rheumatology* 23, no. 6 (2017): 330–39; K. Beyer et al., "Marine Omega-3, Vitamin D Levels, Disease Outcome and Periodontal Status in Rheumatoid Arthritis Outpatients," *Nutrition* 55 (2018): 116–24; CCT Clark et al., "Efficacy of ω-3 Supplementation in Patients with Psoriasis: A Meta-analysis of Randomized Controlled Trials," *Clinical Rheumatology* 38 (2019): 977–88.

51. M. Pedersen et al., "Diet and Risk of Rheumatoid Arthritis in a Prospective Cohort," *Journal of Rheumatology* 32, no. 7 (2005): 1249–52.

52. CN Serhan, "Pro-Resolving Lipid Mediators are Leads for Resolution Physiology," *Nature* 510, no. 7503 (2014): 92–101; I. Zahoor et al., "Specialized Pro-resolving Lipid Mediators: Emerging Therapeutic Candidates for Multiple Sclerosis," *Clinical Reviews in Allergy & Immunology* 60, no. 2 (2021): 147–63; NH Schebb et al., "Formation, Signaling and Occurrence of Specialized Pro-Resolving Lipid Mediators-What Is the Evidence so Far?," *Frontiers in Pharmacology* (2022): 475; A. Val-Blasco et al., "Specialized Proresolving Mediators Protect Against Experimental Autoimmune Myocarditis by Modulating Ca^{2+} Handling and NRF2 Activation," *Basic to Translational Science* 7, no. 6 (2022): 544–60; WA Julliard et al., "Specialized Pro-resolving Mediators as Modulators of Immune Responses," *Seminars in Immunology* (2022): 101605.

53. NA Mesinkovska, "Emerging Unconventional Therapies for Alopecia Areata," *Journal of Investigative Dermatology Symposium Proceedings* 19, no. 1 (2018): S32–S33; Z. Li et al., "Low-Dose Naltrexone (LDN): A Promising Treatment in Immune-Related Diseases and Cancer Therapy," *International Immunopharmacology* 61 (2018): 178–184; KM Bostick et al., "The Use of Low-Dose Naltrexone for Chronic Pain," *Senior Care Pharmacist* 34, no. 1 (2019): 43–46; C. Ekelem et al., "Utility of Naltrexone Treatment for Chronic Inflammatory Dermatologic

Conditions: A Systematic Review," *JAMA Dermatology* 155, no. 2 (2019): 229–36; D. Trofimovitch et al., "Pharmacology Update: Low-Dose Naltrexone as a Possible Nonopioid Modality for Some Chronic, Nonmalignant Pain Syndromes," *American Journal of Hospice and Palliative Medicine* 36, no. 10 (2019): 907–12.

54. N. Sharafaddinzadeh et al., "The Effect of Low-Dose Naltrexone on Quality of Life of Patients with Multiple Sclerosis: A Randomized Placebo-Controlled Trial," *Multiple Sclerosis Journal* 16, no. 8 (2010): 964–69; G. Raknes et al., "Low Dose Naltrexone in Multiple Sclerosis: Effects on Medication Use. A Quasi-Experimental Study," *PLoS One* 12, no. 11 (2017): e0187423; Raknes et al., "Low Dose Naltrexone: Effects on Medication in Rheumatoid and Seropositive Arthritis. A Nationwide Register-Based Controlled Quasi-Experimental Before-After Study," *PLoS One* 14, no. 2 (2019): e0212460; B. Beaudette-Zlatanova et al., "Pilot Study of Low-Dose Naltrexone for the Treatment of Chronic Pain Due to Arthritis: A Randomized, Double-Blind, Placebo-Controlled, Crossover Clinical Trial," *Clinical Therapeutics* (2023).

55. Raknes et al., "Low Dose Naltrexone: Effects on Medication in Rheumatoid and Seropositive Arthritis. A Nationwide Register-Based Controlled Quasi-Experimental Before-After Study," *PLoS One* 14, no. 2 (2019): e0212460.

56. Raknes et al., "No Change in the Consumption of Thyroid Hormones After Starting Low Dose Naltrexone (LDN): A Quasi-Experimental Before-After Study," *BMC Endocrine Disorders* 20 (2020): 1–4; D. Larsen et al., "Thyroid, Diet, and Alternative Approaches," *Journal of Clinical Endocrinology & Metabolism* 107, no. 11 (2022): 2973–81.

57. DC Wraith, "Induction of Antigen-Specific Unresponsiveness with Synthetic Peptides: Specific Immunotherapy for Treatment of Allergic and Autoimmune Conditions," *International Archives of Allergy and Immunology* 108, no. 4 (1995): 355–59; AS Gokhale et al., "Peptides and Peptidomimetics as Immunomodulators," *Immunotherapy* 6, no. 6 (2014): 755–74.

58. DDL Scheffer et al., "Exercise-Induced Immune System Response: Anti-Inflammatory Status on Peripheral and Central Organs," *Biochimica et Biophysica Acta (BBA)-Molecular Basis of Disease* 1866, no. 10 (2020): 165823; J. Wang et al., "Exercise Regulates the Immune System," *Physical Exercise for Human Health* (2020): 395–408.

59. GS Metsios et al., "Exercise and Inflammation," *Best Practice & Research Clinical Rheumatology* 34, no. 2 (2020): 101504.

60. K. Sharif et al., "Physical Activity and Autoimmune Diseases: Get Moving and Manage the Disease," *Autoimmunity Reviews* 17, no. 1 (2018): 53–72; ER Reynolds et al., "Multiple Sclerosis and Exercise: A

Literature Review," *Current Sports Medicine Reports* 17, no. 1 (2018): 31–35; O. Einstein et al., "Physical Exercise Therapy for Autoimmune Neuroinflammation: Application of Knowledge from Animal Models to Patient Care," *Autoimmunity Reviews* 21, no. 4 (2022): 103033.

61. R. Codella et al., "Why Should People with Type 1 Diabetes Exercise Regularly?," *Acta Diabetologica* 54 (2017): 615–30.

62. DB Bartlett et al., "Ten Weeks of High-Intensity Interval Walk Training Is Associated with Reduced Disease Activity and Improved Innate Immune Function in Older Adults with Rheumatoid Arthritis: A Pilot Study," *Arthritis Research & Therapy* 20 (2018): 1–15.

63. AJ Wadley et al., "Preliminary Evidence of Reductive Stress in Human Cytotoxic T Cells Following Exercise," *Journal of Applied Physiology* 125, no. 2 (2018): 586–95.

64. S. Birnbaum et al., "Home-Based Exercise in Autoimmune Myasthenia Gravis: A Randomized Controlled Trial," *Neuromuscular Disorders* 31, no. 8 (2021): 726–35.

65. Merlin Sheldrake, *Entangled Life* (New York: Random House, 2020), 95–96.

66. Mushrooms can help to differentiate CD4+ to "more mature TH1 and TH2 subsets," with a note that autoimmune disease tends to be a TH1 mediated. C. Lull et al., "Antiinflammatory and Immunomodulating Properties of Fungal Metabolites," *Mediators of Inflammation* 2005, no. 2 (2005): 63–80.

Chapter 11: Mind-Body Therapy Protocol

1. SS Dickerson et al., "Immunological Effects of Induced Shame and Guilt," *Psychosomatic Medicine* 66, no. 1 (2004): 124–31.

2. EK Pradhan et al., "Effect of Mindfulness-Based Stress Reduction in Rheumatoid Arthritis Patients," *Arthritis and Rheumatism* 57, no. 7 (2007): 1134–42.

3. M. Daye, "Introduction," in *Hakomi Mindfulness-Centered Somatic Psychotherapy: A Comprehensive Guide to Theory and Practice* (New York: W. W. Norton & Company, 2015), 3.

4. Ibid.

5. M. Mischke-Reeds, "Mindfulness and Trauma States," in *Hakomi Mindfulness-Centered Somatic Psychotherapy: A Comprehensive Guide to Theory and Practice* (New York: W. W. Norton & Company, 2015), 272–80. For more information, go to https://manuelamischkereeds .com.

6. P. Ogden et al., "A Sensorimotor Approach to the Treatment of Trauma and Dissociation," *Psychiatric Clinics* 29, no. 1 (2006): 263–79.

7. DA Monti et al., "Neuro Emotional Technique Effects on Brain

Physiology in Cancer Patients with Traumatic Stress Symptoms: Preliminary Findings," *Journal of Cancer Survivorship* 11 (2017): 438–46.

8. Additional resources for Dr. Monti can be found at https://drdanmonti .com/. DA Monti et al., "Short Term Correlates of the Neuro Emotional Technique for Cancer-Related Traumatic Stress Symptoms: A Pilot Case Series," *Journal of Cancer Survivorship* 1 (2007): 161–66; DA Monti et al., "Changes in Cerebellar Functional Connectivity and Autonomic Regulation in Cancer Patients Treated with the Neuro Emotional Technique for Traumatic Stress Symptoms," *Journal of Cancer Survivorship* 12 (2018): 145–53.

9. In the twelve traditions of twelve-step programs, we follow the principle of anonymity. Learn more at https://www.aa.org/. See also B. Wilson, *Alcoholics Anonymous: The Big Book* (United States: Must Have Books, 2021).

10. A. Hill, "LSD Could Help Alcoholics Stop Drinking, AA Founder Believed," *The Guardian*, August 2012, https://www.theguardian.com/ science/2012/aug/23/lsd-help-alcoholics-theory.

11. SW Porges, "The Polyvagal Perspective," *Biological Psychology* 74, no. 2 (2007): 116–43; SW Porges, "The Polyvagal Theory: New Insights into Adaptive Reactions of the Autonomic Nervous System," *Cleveland Clinic Journal of Medicine* 76, no. 2 (2009): S86; SW Porges et al., "The Early Development of the Autonomic Nervous System Provides a Neural Platform for Social Behavior: A Polyvagal Perspective," *Infant and Child Development* 20, no. 1 (2011): 106–18; J. Kolacz et al., "Traumatic Stress and the Autonomic Brain-Gut Connection in Development: Polyvagal Theory as an Integrative Framework for Psychosocial and Gastrointestinal Pathology," *Developmental Psychobiology* 61, no. 5 (2019): 796–809; SW Porges, "Polyvagal Theory: A Science of Safety," *Frontiers in Integrative Neuroscience* 16 (2022): 27; JS Doody et al., "The Evolution of Sociality and the Polyvagal Theory," *Biological Psychology* (2023): 108569.

Chapter 12: Everything You Want to Know About Psychedelics

1. MW Johnson et al., "Classic Psychedelics: An Integrative Review of Epidemiology, Therapeutics, Mystical Experience, and Brain Network Function," *Pharmacology & Therapeutics* 197 (2019): 83–102.

2. I. Magaraggia et al., "Improving Cognitive Functioning in Major Depressive Disorder with Psychedelics: A Dimensional Approach," *Neurobiology of Learning and Memory* 183 (2021): 107467; H. Gill et al., "The Effects of Psilocybin in Adults with Major Depressive Disorder and the General Population: Findings from Neuroimaging

Studies," *Psychiatry Research* (2022): 114577; AE Calder et al., "Towards an Understanding of Psychedelic-Induced Neuroplasticity," *Neuropsychopharmacology* 48, no. 1 (2023): 104–12.

3. GM Knudsen, "Sustained Effects of Single Doses of Classical Psychedelics in Humans," *Neuropsychopharmacology* 48, no. 1 (2023): 145–50.

4. SP Cohen et al., "Consensus Guidelines on the Use of Intravenous Ketamine Infusions for Chronic Pain from the American Society of Regional Anesthesia and Pain Medicine, the American Academy of Pain Medicine, and the American Society of Anesthesiologists," *Regional Anesthesia & Pain Medicine* 43, no. 5 (2018): 521–46; V. Orhurhu et al., "Ketamine Infusions for Chronic Pain: A Systematic Review and Meta-analysis of Randomized Controlled Trials," *Anesthesia & Analgesia* 129, no. 1 (2019): 241–54; A. Corriger et al., "Ketamine and Depression: A Narrative Review," *Drug Design, Development and Therapy* (2019): 3051–67; A. Bahji et al., "Comparative Efficacy of Racemic Ketamine and Esketamine for Depression: A Systematic Review and Meta-Analysis," *Journal of Affective Disorders* 278 (2021): 542–55; LA Jelen et al., "Ketamine for Depression," *International Review of Psychiatry* 33, no. 3 (2021): 207–28; G. Martinotti et al., "Therapeutic Potentials of Ketamine and Esketamine in Obsessive-Compulsive Disorder (OCD), Substance Use Disorders (SUD) and Eating Disorders (ED): A Review of the Current Literature," *Brain Sciences* 11, no. 7 (2021): 856; M. Abbar et al., "Ketamine for the Acute Treatment of Severe Suicidal Ideation: Double Blind, Randomised Placebo Controlled Trial," *BMJ* 376 (2022); A. Ragnhildstveit et al., "Ketamine as a Novel Psychopharmacotherapy for Eating Disorders: Evidence and Future Directions," *Brain Sciences* 12, no. 3 (2022): 382; M. Voute et al., "Ketamine in Chronic Pain: A Delphi Survey," *European Journal of Pain* 26, no. 4 (2022): 873–87.

5. JM Mitchell et al., "MDMA-Assisted Therapy for Severe PTSD: A Randomized, Double-Blind, Placebo-Controlled Phase 3 Study," *Nature Medicine* 27, no. 6 (2021): 1025–33; KW Smith et al., "MDMA-Assisted Psychotherapy for Treatment of Posttraumatic Stress Disorder: A Systematic Review with Meta-Analysis," *Journal of Clinical Pharmacology* 62, no. 4 (2022): 463–71.

6. S. Muttoni et al., "Classical Psychedelics for the Treatment of Depression and Anxiety: A Systematic Review," *Journal of Affective Disorders* 258 (2019): 11–24; D. De Gregorio et al., "Hallucinogens in Mental Health: Preclinical and Clinical Studies on LSD, Psilocybin, MDMA, and Ketamine," *Journal of Neuroscience* 41, no. 5 (2021): 891–900; P. Oehen et al., "Using a MDMA- and LSD-Group Therapy Model

in Clinical Practice in Switzerland and Highlighting the Treatment of Trauma-Related Disorders," *Frontiers in Psychiatry* (2022): 739.

7. WN Pahnke et al., "LSD Assisted Psychotherapy with Terminal Cancer Patients," *Current Psychiatric Therapies* 9 (1969): 144–52; S. Grof et al., "LSD-Assisted Psychotherapy in Patients with Terminal Cancer," *International Pharmacopsychiatry* 8 (1973): 129–44; RC Clyman, "LSD Psychotherapy: A Review of the Literature and Some Proposals for Future Research," *Rhode Island Medical Journal* 55, no. 9 (1972): 282–86; AA Kurland, "LSD in the Supportive Care of the Terminally Ill Cancer Patient," *Journal of Psychoactive Drugs* 17, no. 4 (1985): 279–90; M. Winkelman, "Psychedelics as Medicines for Substance Abuse Rehabilitation: Evaluating Treatments with LSD, Peyote, Ibogaine and Ayahuasca," *Current Drug Abuse Reviews* 7, no. 2 (2014): 101–16; ME Liechti, "Modern Clinical Research on LSD," *Neuropsychopharmacology: Official Publication of the American College of Neuropsychopharmacology* 42, no. 11 (2017), 2114–27; DE Nichols, "Dark Classics in Chemical Neuroscience: Lysergic Acid Diethylamide (LSD)," *ACS Chemical Neuroscience* 9, no. 10 (2018): 2331–43; S. Muttoni et al., "Classical Psychedelics for the Treatment of Depression and Anxiety: A Systematic Review," *Journal of Affective Disorders* 258 (2019): 11–24; D. De Gregorio et al., "Repeated Lysergic Acid Diethylamide (LSD) Reverses Stress-Induced Anxiety-Like Behavior, Cortical Synaptogenesis Deficits and Serotonergic Neurotransmission Decline," *Neuropsychopharmacology* 47, no. 6 (2022): 1188–98; H. Lowe et al., "Psychedelics: Alternative and Potential Therapeutic Options for Treating Mood and Anxiety Disorders," *Molecules* 27, no. 8 (2022): 2520.

8. WN Pahnke et al., "The Experimental Use of Psychedelic (LSD) Psychotherapy," *JAMA* 212, no. 11 (1970): 1856–63.

9. Y. Celidwen et al., "Ethical Principles of Traditional Indigenous Medicine to Guide Western Psychedelic Research and Practice," *Lancet Regional Health—Americas* 18 (2023): 100410.

10. DE Gard et al., "Evaluating the Risk of Psilocybin for the Treatment of Bipolar Depression: A Review of the Research Literature and Published Case Studies," *Journal of Affective Disorders Reports* 6 (December 2021): 1002240.

11. FA Moreno et al., "Safety, Tolerability, and Efficacy of Psilocybin in 9 Patients with Obsessive-Compulsive Disorder," *Journal of Clinical Psychiatry* 67, no. 11 (2006): 1735–40; MP Bogenschutz et al., "Psilocybin-Assisted Treatment for Alcohol Dependence: A Proof-of-Concept Study," *Journal of Psychopharmacology* 29, no. 3 (2015): 289–99; H. Castro Santos et al., "What Is the Clinical Evidence on Psilocybin for the Treatment of Psychiatric Disorders?

A Systematic Review," *Porto Biomedical Journal* 6, no. 1 (2021); KAA Andersen et al., "Therapeutic Effects of Classic Serotonergic Psychedelics: A Systematic Review of Modern-Era Clinical Studies," *Acta Psychiatrica Scandinavica* 143, no. 2 (2021): 101–18; S. Ling et al., "Molecular Mechanisms of Psilocybin and Implications for the Treatment of Depression," *CNS Drugs* 36, no. 1 (2022): 17–30; H. Gill et al., "The Effects of Psilocybin in Adults with Major Depressive Disorder and the General Population: Findings from Neuroimaging Studies," *Psychiatry Research* (2022): 114577; MP Bogenschutz et al., "Percentage of Heavy Drinking Days Following Psilocybin-Assisted Psychotherapy vs Placebo in the Treatment of Adult Patients with Alcohol Use Disorder: A Randomized Clinical Trial," *JAMA Psychiatry* 79, no. 10 (2022): 953–62; Y. Celidwen et al., "Ethical Principles of Traditional Indigenous Medicine to Guide Western Psychedelic Research and Practice," *Lancet Regional Health—Americas* 18 (2023): 100410; MI Husain et al., "Serotonergic Psychedelics for Depression: What Do We Know About Neurobiological Mechanisms of Action?," *Frontiers in Psychiatry* 13 (2022).

12. T. White, "Falling for Psychedelics," *Stanford Magazine*, March 2023, https://stanfordmag.org/contents/falling-for-psychedelics; S. Marwaha et al., "Novel and Emerging Treatments for Major Depression," *The Lancet* 401, no. 10371 (2023): 141–53.

13. J. Bornemann et al., "Self-Medication for Chronic Pain Using Classic Psychedelics: A Qualitative Investigation to Inform Future Research," *Frontiers in Psychiatry* 12 (2021): 735427; "Dr. Robin Carhart-Harris: The Science of Psychedelics for Mental Health," Huberman Lab, May 22, 2023, https://hubermanlab.com/dr-robin-carhart-harris-the-science-of-psychedelics-for-mental-health/.

14. AL Harvey et al., "Pharmacological Actions of the South African Medicinal and Functional Food Plant Sceletium Tortuosum and Its Principal Alkaloids," *Journal of Ethnopharmacology* 137, no. 3 (2011): 1124–29; MC Manganyi et al., "A Chewable Cure "Kanna": Biological and Pharmaceutical Properties of *Sceletium Tortuosum*," *Molecules* 26, no. 9 (2021): 2557.

15. JL Krstenansky, "Mesembrine Alkaloids: Review of Their Occurrence, Chemistry, and Pharmacology," *Journal of Ethnopharmacology* 195 (2017): 10–19; J. Reay Jet al., "Sceletium Tortuosum (Zembrin®) Ameliorates Experimentally Induced Anxiety in Healthy Volunteers," *Human Psychopharmacology: Clinical and Experimental* 35, no. 6 (2020): 1–7; K. Reddy et al., "Mass Spectrometry Metabolomics and Feature-Based Molecular Networking Reveals Population-Specific Chemistry in Some Species of the *Sceletium* Genus," *Frontiers in Nutrition* 9 (2022);

OJ Onaolapo et al., "Substance Use and Substance Use Disorders in Africa: An Epidemiological Approach to the Review of Existing Literature," *World Journal of Psychiatry* 12, no. 10 (2022): 1268–86.

16. N. Gericke et al., "Sceletium—A Review Update," *Journal of Ethnopharmacology* 119, no. 3 (2008): 653–63; AC Bennett et al., "Sceletium Tortuosum May Delay Chronic Disease Progression Via Alkaloid-Dependent Antioxidant or Anti-Inflammatory Action," *Journal of Physiology and Biochemistry* 74 (2018): 539–47; TL Olatunji et al., "Sceletium Tortuosum: A Review on Its Phytochemistry, Pharmacokinetics, Biological and Clinical Activities," *Journal of Ethnopharmacology* 280 (2021): 114476.

17. WebMD, "Sceletium—Uses, Side Effects, and More," https://www.webmd.com/vitamins/ai/ingredientmono-1259/sceletium.

18. D. McQueen, *Psychedelic Cannabis: Therapeutic Methods and Unique Blends to Treat Trauma and Transform Consciousness* (Rochester, VT: Inner Traditions/Bear & Company, 2021).

19. "Executive function" refers to the activity of multiple cognitive processes that allow you to anticipate consequences, set and follow goals, and experience self-control—and serotonin signaling at the serotonin 2A receptors is key with the prefrontal cortex (your brain's CEO) as the main agent. The lateral septal nucleus is one of the most strategically important positions in the forebrain, because it connects the structures of the limbic system with different sites of the brain stem. S. Aznar et al., "Regulating Prefrontal Cortex Activation: An Emerging Role for the 5-HT$_2$A Serotonin Receptor in the Modulation of Emotion-Based Actions?," *Molecular Neurobiology* 48 (2013): 841–53, DO Borroto-Escuela et al., "Hallucinogenic 5-HT2AR Agonists LSD and DOI Enhance Dopamine D2R Protomer Recognition and Signaling of D2-5-HT2A Heteroreceptor Complexes," *Biochemical and Biophysical Research Communications* 443, no. 1 (2014): 278–84; G. Zhang et al., "The Role of Serotonin 5-HT2A Receptors in Memory and Cognition," *Frontiers in Pharmacology* 6 (2015): 225; S. Aznar et al., "The 5-HT2A Serotonin Receptor in Executive Function: Implications for Neuropsychiatric and Neurodegenerative Diseases," *Neuroscience & Biobehavioral Reviews* 64 (2016): 63–82; G. Zhang et al., "Examination of the Hippocampal Contribution to Serotonin 5-HT2A Receptor-Mediated Facilitation of Object Memory in C57BL/6J Mice," *Neuropharmacology* 109 (2016): 332–40; A. García-Bea et al., "Serotonin 5-HT$_{2A}$ Receptor Expression and Functionality in Postmortem Frontal Cortex of Subjects with Schizophrenia: Selective Biased Agonism via G$_{\alpha i1}$-Proteins," *European Neuropsychopharmacology* 29, no. 12 (2019): 1453–63; AB Casey et

al., "'Selective' Serotonin 5-HT$_{2A}$ Receptor Antagonists," *Biochemical Pharmacology* (2022): 115028.

20. AE Calder et al., "Towards an Understanding of Psychedelic-Induced Neuroplasticity," *Neuropsychopharmacology* 48, no. 1 (2023):104–12.

21. I. Magaraggia et al., "Improving Cognitive Functioning in Major Depressive Disorder with Psychedelics: A Dimensional Approach," *Neurobiology of Learning and Memory* 183 (2021): 107467.

22. Betty Eisner was a psychologist who pioneered use of psychedelic drugs to augment psychotherapy, including LSD. Her care was revolutionary but also triggered one or more investigations by the Board of Medical Quality Assurance of California.

23. See Daniel McQueen's "Set, Setting, Skill," accessed May 30, 2023, https://psychedelicsittersschool.org/about-the-center-for-medicinal-mindfulness/.

24. See Jasmine Virdi and Dr. Kwasi Adusei on their use of "Support" in preparation, accessed May 30, 2023, https://psychedelicstoday .com/2022/12/21/thinking-beyond-set-and-setting-in-the-psychedelic-experience/.

25. F. Holze et al., "Direct Comparison of the Acute Effects of Lysergic Acid Diethylamide and Psilocybin in a Double-Blind Placebo-Controlled Study in Healthy Subjects," *Neuropsychopharmacology* 47 (2022): 1180–87.

26. NRPW Hutten et al., "Low Doses of LSD Acutely Increase BDNF Blood Plasma Levels in Healthy Volunteers," *ACS Pharmacology & Translational Science* 4, no. 2 (2020): 461–66.

27. J. Fadiman et al., "Might Microdosing Psychedelics Be Safe and Beneficial? An Initial Exploration," *Journal of Psychoactive Drugs* 51, no. 2 (2019): 118–22; NRPW Hutten et al., "Low Doses of LSD Acutely Increase BDNF Blood Plasma Levels in Healthy Volunteers," *ACS Pharmacology & Translational Science* 4, no. 2 (2020): 461–66. Mitchell JM et al., "MDMA-Assisted Therapy for Severe PTSD: A Randomized, Double-Blind, Placebo-Controlled Phase 3 Study," *Focus* (Am Psychiatry Publication). 2023 21, no. 3:315-328.

28. T. Lea et al., "Microdosing Psychedelics: Motivations, Subjective Effects and Harm Reduction," *International Journal of Drug Policy* 75 (2020): 102600.

29. DE Olson, "Psychoplastogens: A Promising Class of Plasticity-Promoting Neurotherapeutics," *Journal of Experimental Neuroscience* 12 (2018): 1179069518800508; AC Kaypak et al., "Macrodosing to Microdosing with Psychedelics: Clinical, Social, and Cultural Perspectives," *Transcultural Psychiatry* 59, no. 5 (2022): 665–74.

30. JM Rootman et al., "Psilocybin Microdosers Demonstrate Greater Observed Improvements in Mood and Mental Health at One Month Relative to Non-Microdosing Controls," *Scientific Reports* 12, no. 1 (2022): 11091.

31. R. Petranker et al., "Microdosing Psychedelics: Subjective Benefits and Challenges, Substance Testing Behavior, and the Relevance of Intention," *Journal of Psychopharmacology* 36, no. 1 (2022): 85–96.

32. T. Anderson et al., "Psychedelic Microdosing Benefits and Challenges: An Empirical Codebook," *Harm Reduction Journal* 16, no. 1 (2019): 1–10.

33. KP Kuypers et al., "Microdosing Psychedelics: More Questions Than Answers? An Overview and Suggestions for Future Research," *Journal of Psychopharmacology* 33, no. 9 (2019): 1039–57.

34. J. Marschall et al., "Psilocybin Microdosing Does Not Affect Emotion-Related Symptoms and Processing: A Preregistered Field and Lab-Based Study," *Journal of Psychopharmacology* 36, no. 1 (2022): 97–113.

35. KP Kuypers, "The Therapeutic Potential of Microdosing Psychedelics in Depression," *Therapeutic Advances in Psychopharmacology* 10 (2020): 2045125320950567.

36. B. Szigeti et al., "Self-blinding Citizen Science to Explore Psychedelic Microdosing," *Elife* 10 (2021): e62878; V. Polito et al., "The Emerging Science of Microdosing: A Systematic Review of Research on Low Dose Psychedelics (1955–2021) and Recommendations for the Field," *Neuroscience & Biobehavioral Reviews* (2022): 104706.

37. T. Anderson et al., "Microdosing Psychedelics: Personality, Mental Health, and Creativity Differences in Microdosers," *Psychopharmacology* 236 (2019): 731–40.

38. NRPW Hutten et al., "Self-Rated Effectiveness of Microdosing with Psychedelics for Mental and Physical Health Problems Among Microdosers," *Frontiers in Psychiatry* 10 (2019): 672; G. Ona et al., "Potential Safety, Benefits, and Influence of the Placebo Effect in Microdosing Psychedelic Drugs: A Systematic Review," *Neuroscience & Biobehavioral Reviews* 119 (2020): 194–203; LP Cameron, "Asking Questions of Psychedelic Microdosing," *Elife* 10 (2021): e66920; V. Hartong et al., "Psychedelic Microdosing, Mindfulness, and Anxiety: A Cross-Sectional Mediation Study," *Journal of Psychoactive Drugs* (2022): 1–11; A. Wong et al., "Microdosing with Classical Psychedelics: Research Trajectories and Practical Considerations," *Transcultural Psychiatry* 59, no. 5 (2022): 675–90.

39. B. Huber, "What Do We Know About the Risks of Psychedelics?," Michael Pollan, https://michaelpollan.com/psychedelics-risk-today/.

40. See "Most Harmful Drugs" graph in "Alcohol 'More Harmful Than

Heroin' Says Prof David Nutt," BBC, November 1, 2010, https://www.bbc.com/news/uk-11660210.

41. DE Gard et al., "Evaluating the Risk of Psilocybin for the Treatment of Bipolar Depression: A Review of the Research Literature and Published Case Studies," *Journal of Affective Disorders Reports* 6 (December 2021): 1002240.

42. AK Schlag et al., "Adverse Effects of Psychedelics: From Anecdotes and Misinformation to Systematic Science," *Journal of Psychopharmacology* 36, no. 2 (2022): 258–72.

43. B. Malcolm et al., "Serotonin Toxicity of Serotonergic Psychedelics," *Psychopharmacology* 239, no. 6 (2022): 1881–91.

44. PA Frewen et al., "Toward a Psychobiology of Posttraumatic Self-Dysregulation: Reexperiencing, Hyperarousal, Dissociation, and Emotional Numbing," *Annals of the New York Academy of Sciences* 1071, no. 1 (2006): 110–24.

45. SK Kamboj et al., "Recreational 3,4-methylenedioxy-N-methylamphetamine (MDMA) or 'Ecstasy' and Self-Focused Compassion: Preliminary Steps in the Development of a Therapeutic Psychopharmacology of Contemplative Practices," *Journal of Psychopharmacology* 29, no. 9 (2015): 961–70.

46. G. Bedi et al.," Effects of MDMA on Sociability and Neural Response to Social Threat and Social Reward," *Psychopharmacology* 207 (2009): 73–83; CM Hysek et al., "MDMA Enhances Emotional Empathy and Prosocial Behavior," *Social Cognitive and Affective Neuroscience* 9, no. 11 (2014): 1645–52; SM Keller et al., "Understanding Factors Associated with Early Therapeutic Alliance in PTSD Treatment: Adherence, Childhood Sexual Abuse History, and Social Support," *Journal of Consulting and Clinical Psychology* 78, no. 6 (2010): 974; ZE Imel et al., "Meta-Analysis of Dropout in Treatments for Posttraumatic Stress Disorder," *Journal of Consulting and Clinical Psychology* 81, no. 3 (2013): 394; M. Mithoefer, "MDMA-Assisted Psychotherapy; Promising Treatment for PTSD," American Psychiatric Association Annual Meeting (2015).

47. JM Mitchell et al., "MDMA-Assisted Therapy for Severe PTSD: A Randomized, Double-Blind, Placebo-Controlled Phase 3 Study," *Nature Medicine* 27, no. 6 (2021): 1025–33.

48. NT Boyle et al., "Methylenedioxymethamphetamine ('Ecstasy')-Induced Immunosuppression: A Cause for Concern?," *British Journal of Pharmacology* 161, no. 1 (2010): 17–32.

49. MC Mithoefer et al., "MDMA-Assisted Psychotherapy for Treatment of PTSD: Study Design and Rationale for Phase 3 Trials Based on Pooled Analysis of Six Phase 2 Randomized Controlled Trials,"

Psychopharmacology 236 (2019): 2735–45; R. Nardou et al., "Oxytocin-Dependent Reopening of a Social Reward Learning Critical Period with MDMA," *Nature* 569, no. 7754 (2019): 116–20.

50. FX Vollenweider et al., "Classic Psychedelic Drugs: Update on Biological Mechanisms," *Pharmacopsychiatry* 55, no. 3 (2022): 121–38.

51. CE Canal, "Serotonergic Psychedelics: Experimental Approaches for Assessing Mechanisms of Action," *Handbook of Experimental Pharmacology* 252 (2018): 227–60; FS Barrett et al., "Psilocybin Acutely Alters the Functional Connectivity of the Claustrum with Brain Networks that Support Perception, Memory, and Attention," *Neuroimage* 218 (2020): 116980; JJ Gattuso et al., "Default Mode Network Modulation by Psychedelics: A Systematic Review," *International Journal of Neuropsychopharmacology* 26, no. 3 (2023): 155–88.

52. See the helpful lecture on healing states of consciousness by Brad Jacobs, MD, "Psychedelic Medicine—Next Frontier in Mental Health," YouTube, https://youtu.be/Fr8r96s37ys.

Chapter 13: Your Autoimmune Blueprint

1. VJ Felitti et al., "Relationship of Childhood Abuse and Household Dysfunction to Many of the Leading Causes of Death in Adults: The Adverse Childhood Experiences (ACE) Study," *American Journal of Preventive Medicine* 14, no. 4 (1998): 245–58; S. Su et al., "Adverse Childhood Experiences Are Associated with Detrimental Hemodynamics and Elevated Circulating Endothelin-1 in Adolescents and Young Adults," *Hypertension* 64, no. 1 (2014): 201–7; W. Akosile et al., "The Association Between Post-Traumatic Stress Disorder and Coronary Artery Disease: A Meta-Analysis," *Australasian Psychiatry* 26, no. 5 (2018): 524–30; A. Basu et al., "Childhood Maltreatment and Health Impact: The Examples of Cardiovascular Disease and Type 2 Diabetes Mellitus in Adults," *Clinical Psychology: Science and Practice* 24, no. 2 (2017): 125; A. Tawakol et al., "Relation Between Resting Amygdalar Activity and Cardiovascular Events: A Longitudinal and Cohort Study," *The Lancet* 389, no. 10071 (2017): 834–45; LC Godoy et al., "Association of Adverse Childhood Experiences with Cardiovascular Disease Later in Life: A Review," *JAMA Cardiology* 6, no. 2 (2021): 228–35; NDM Jenkins et al., "Childhood Psychosocial Stress Is Linked with Impaired Vascular Endothelial Function, Lower SIRT1, and Oxidative Stress in Young Adulthood," *American Journal of Physiology-Heart and Circulatory Physiology* 321, no. 3 (2021): H532–41; P. Rodriguez-Miguelez et al., "The Link Between Childhood Adversity and Cardiovascular Disease Risk: Role of Cerebral and Systemic Vasculature,"

Function (2022); NDM Jenkins et al., "How Do Adverse Childhood Experiences Get Under the Skin to Promote Cardiovascular Disease? A Focus on Vascular Health," *Function* 3, no. 4 (2022): zqac032; S. Mrug et al., "Early Life Stress, Coping, and Cardiovascular Reactivity to Acute Social Stress," *Psychosomatic Medicine* 85, no. 2 (2023): 118–29; R. de la Rosa et al., "Biological Burden of Adverse Childhood Experiences in Children," *Psychosomatic Medicine* 85, no. 2 (2023): 108–17.

2. C. Kreatsoulas et al., "Young Adults and Adverse Childhood Events: A Potent Measure of Cardiovascular Risk," *American Journal of Medicine* 132, no. 5 (2019): 605–13; L. Lin et al., "Adverse Childhood Experiences and Subsequent Chronic Diseases Among Middle-Aged or Older Adults in China and Associations with Demographic and Socioeconomic Characteristics," *JAMA Network Open* 4, no. 10 (2021): e2130143.

3. K. Wingenfeld et al., "Are Adverse Childhood Experiences and Depression Associated with Impaired Glucose Tolerance in Females? An Experimental Study," *Journal of Psychiatric Research* 95 (2017): 60–67; SS Deschênes et al., "Adverse Childhood Experiences and the Risk of Diabetes: Examining the Roles of Depressive Symptoms and Cardiometabolic Dysregulations in the Whitehall II Cohort Study," *Diabetes Care* 41, no. 10 (2018): 2120–26; V. Jimenez et al., "Associations of Adverse Childhood Experiences with Stress Physiology and Insulin Resistance in Adolescents at Risk for Adult Obesity," *Developmental Psychobiology* 63, no. 6 (2021): e22127; M. Kivimäki et al., "The Multiple Roles of Life Stress in Metabolic Disorders," *Nature Reviews Endocrinology* 19, no. 1 (2023): 10–27.

4. C. Muniz Carvalho et al., "Dissecting the Genetic Association of C-Reactive Protein with PTSD, Traumatic Events, and Social Support," *Neuropsychopharmacology* 46, no. 6 (2021): 1071–77.

5. A. O'Neil et al., "Gender/Sex as a Social Determinant of Cardiovascular Risk," *Circulation* 137, no. 8 (2018): 854–64; C. Meinhausen et al., "Posttraumatic Stress Disorder (PTSD), Sleep, and Cardiovascular Disease Risk: A Mechanism-Focused Narrative Review," *Health Psychology* 41, no. 10 (2022): 663; W. Akosile et al., "Genetic Correlation and Causality Assessment Between Post-Traumatic Stress Disorder and Coronary Artery Disease-Related Traits," *Gene* 842 (2022): 146802; R. Polimanti et al., "Understanding the Comorbidity Between Posttraumatic Stress Severity and Coronary Artery Disease Using Genome-Wide Information and Electronic Health Records," *Molecular Psychiatry* (2022): 1–9; JA Sumner et al., "Psychological and Biological Mechanisms Linking Trauma with Cardiovascular Disease Risk," *Translational Psychiatry* 13, no. 1 (2023): 25.

6. S. Danese et al., "Immune Regulation by Microvascular Endothelial Cells: Directing Innate and Adaptive Immunity, Coagulation, and Inflammation," *Journal of Immunology* 178, no. 10 (2007): 6017–22; S. Sitia et al., "From Endothelial Dysfunction to Atherosclerosis," *Autoimmunity Reviews* 9, no. 12 (2010): 830–34; S. Su et al., "Adverse Childhood Experiences are Associated with Detrimental Hemodynamics and Elevated Circulating Endothelin-1 in Adolescents and Young Adults," *Hypertension* 64, no. 1 (2014): 201–7; RE Konst et al., "The Pathogenic Role of Coronary Microvascular Dysfunction in the Setting of Other Cardiac or Systemic Conditions," *Cardiovascular Research* 116, no. 4 (2020): 817–28; T. Chaikijurajai et al., "Myeloperoxidase: A Potential Therapeutic Target for Coronary Artery Disease," *Expert Opinion on Therapeutic Targets* 24, no. 7 (2020): 695–705; NJ Montarello et al., "Inflammation in Coronary Atherosclerosis and Its Therapeutic Implications," *Cardiovascular Drugs and Therapy* (2020): 1–16; G. Markousis-Mavrogenis et al., "Coronary Microvascular Disease: The 'Meeting Point' of Cardiology, Rheumatology and Endocrinology," *European Journal of Clinical Investigation* 52, no. 5 (2022): e13737.

7. I. Hollan et al., "Cardiovascular Disease in Autoimmune Rheumatic Diseases," *Autoimmunity Reviews* 12, no. 10 (2013): 1004–15; J. Ahearn et al., "Cardiovascular Disease Biomarkers Across Autoimmune Diseases," *Clinical Immunology* 161, no. 1 (2015): 59–63; VL Wolf et al., "Autoimmune Disease-Associated Hypertension," *Current Hypertension Reports* 21 (2019): 1–9; M. Gawałko et al., "Cardiac Arrhythmias in Autoimmune Diseases," *Circulation Journal* 84, no. 5 (2020): 685–94; KA Kott et al., "Single-Cell Immune Profiling in Coronary Artery Disease: The Role of State-of-the-Art Immunophenotyping with Mass Cytometry in the Diagnosis of Atherosclerosis," *Journal of the American Heart Association* 9, no. 24 (2020): e017759; M. Casian et al., "Cardiovascular Disease in Primary Sjögren's Syndrome: Raising Clinicians' Awareness," *Frontiers in Immunology* (2022): 2721; S. Onuora, "Autoimmune Disease Increases CVD Risk," *Nature Reviews Rheumatology* 18, no. 11 (2022): 612.

8. "Loneliness in America," Cigna Group, accessed May 28, 2023, https://newsroom.thecignagroup.com/loneliness-in-america.

9. Read more about Brad Jacobs, MD, a concierge and integrative physician and TEDx speaker at https://www.bluewavemedicine.com/.

10. BJ Fogg, *Tiny Habits: The Small Changes That Change Everything* (Boston: Houghton Mifflin Harcourt, 2020).

RESOURCES

Recommended Books

PSYCHEDELIC

CM Bache. *LSD and the Mind of the Universe: Diamonds from Heaven* (New York: Simon & Schuster, 2019).

J. Fadiman. *The Psychedelic Explorer's Guide: Safe, Therapeutic, and Sacred Journeys* (New York: Simon & Schuster, 2011).

S. Grof. *LSD: Doorway to the Numinous: The Groundbreaking Psychedelic Research into Realms of the Human Unconscious* (Ukraine: Inner Traditions/Bear, 2009).

S. Grof. *LSD Psychotherapy: The Healing Potential of Psychedelic Medicine* (San Jose, CA: MAPS, 2008).

S. Grof. *Psychology of the Future: Lessons from Modern Consciousness Research* (Albany, NY: State University of New York Press, 2019).

S. Grof. *Realms of the Human Unconscious: Observations from LSD Research* (London: Souvenir Press, 2016).

S. Grof. *The Way of the Psychonaut: Encyclopedia for Inner Journeys*, vols. 1 and 2 (San Jose, CA: MAPS, 2019).

S. Grof et al. *Holotropic Breathwork: A New Approach to Self-Exploration and Therapy* (Albany, NY: State University of New York Press, 2010).

M. Pollan. *How to Change Your Mind: The New Science of Psychedelics* (New York: Penguin Books Limited, 2018).

M. Pollan. *This Is Your Mind on Plants* (New York: Penguin Press, 2021).

J. Tafur. *The Fellowship of the River: A Medical Doctor's Exploration into Traditional Amazonian Plant Medicine* (Phoenix: Espiritu Books, 2017).

HEALTH

S. Ballantyne. *The Paleo Approach Cookbook: A Detailed Guide to Heal Your Body and Nourish Your Soul* (Nicaragua: Victory Belt Publishing, 2014).

S. Ballantyne. *The Paleo Approach: Reverse Autoimmune Disease and Heal Your Body* (Las Vegas: Victory Belt Publishing, 2014).

S. Ballantyne. *Paleo Principles: The Science Behind the Paleo Template, Step-by-Step Guides, Meal Plans, and 200 + Healthy & Delicious Recipes for Real Life* (Las Vegas: Victory Belt Publishing, 2017).

A. Christianson. *The Adrenal Reset Diet: Strategically Cycle Carbs and Proteins to Lose Weight, Balance Hormones, and Move from Stressed to Thriving* (New York: Rodale, 2014).

A. Christianson. *Healing Hashimoto's: A Savvy Patient's Guide* (Scotts Valley, CA: CreateSpace Independent Publishing Platform, 2012).

A. Christianson. *The Hormone Healing Cookbook: 80+ Recipes to Balance Hormones and Treat Fatigue, Brain Fog, Insomnia, and More* (New York: Rodale, 2023).

A. Christianson. *The Metabolism Reset Diet: Repair Your Liver, Stop Storing Fat and Lose Weight Naturally* (Carlsbad, CA: Hay House, 2019).

A. Christianson. *The Thyroid Reset Diet: Reverse Hypothyroidism and Hashimoto's Symptoms with a Proven Iodine-Balancing Plan* (New York: Rodale, 2021).

A. Christianson et al. *The Complete Idiot's Guide to Thyroid Disease* (New York: DK Publishing, 2011).

A. Christianson et al. *Take Charge of Your Thyroid Disorder: Learn What's Causing Your Hashimoto's Thyroiditis, Graves' Disease, Goiters, Thyroid Nodules, or Other Thyroid Disorders—And What You Can Do About It* (New York: DK, 2020).

BJ Fogg. *Tiny Habits: The Small Changes That Change Everything* (Boston: Houghton Mifflin Harcourt, 2019).

D. Hartwig et al. *The Whole30: The 30-Day Guide to Total Health and Food Freedom* (Boston: Houghton Mifflin Harcourt, 2015).

J. Kabat-Zinn. *Mindfulness Meditation for Pain Relief: Practices to Reclaim Your Body and Your Life* (Louisville, CO: Sounds True, 2023).

V. Longo. *The Longevity Diet: Slow Aging, Fight Disease, Optimize Weight* (New York: Penguin Publishing Group, 2019).

DA Monti et al. *Brain Weaver: Creating the Fabric for a Healthy Mind Through Integrative Medicine* (New York: W. W. Norton & Company, 2021).

DA Monti et al. *Tapestry of Health: Weaving Wellness into Your Life Through the New Science of Integrative Medicine* (New York: W. W. Norton & Company, 2020).

A. Palanisamy. *The TIGER Protocol: An Integrative, 5-Step Program to Treat and Heal Your Autoimmunity* (New York: Grand Central Publishing, 2023).

R. Schwartz. *No Bad Parts: Healing Trauma and Restoring Wholeness with the Internal Family Systems Model* (Louisville, CO: Sounds True, 2021).

T. Wahls. *Minding My Mitochondria: How I Overcame Secondary Progressive Multiple Sclerosis (MS) and Got Out of My Wheelchair* (Germany: TZ Press, 2010).

T. Wahls et al. *The Wahls Protocol Cooking for Life: The Revolutionary Modern Paleo Plan to Treat All Chronic Autoimmune Conditions* (New York: Penguin Publishing Group, 2017).

T. Wahls et al. *The Wahls Protocol: How I Beat Progressive MS Using Paleo Principles and Functional Medicine* (New York: Penguin Publishing Group, 2014).

GENERAL INTEREST

EN Aron. *The Highly Sensitive Person: How to Thrive When the World Overwhelms You* (New York: Citadel Press, 2013).

L. Rankin. *Sacred Medicine: A Doctor's Quest to Unravel the Mysteries of Healing* (Louisville, CO: Sounds True, 2024).

K. Sheppard. *Food Addiction: The Body Knows: Revised & Expanded Edition by Kay Sheppard* (Deerfield Beach, FL: Health Communications, Inc., 2010).

B. Wilson. *Alcoholics Anonymous: The Big Book* (United States: Must Have Books, 2021).

TRAUMA

P. Conti. *Trauma: The Invisible Epidemic: How Trauma Works and How We Can Heal from It* (London: Ebury Publishing, 2022).

G. Johanson et al. *Hakomi Mindfulness Centered Somatic Psychotherapy: A Comprehensive Guide to Theory and Practice* (London: W. W. Norton & Company, 2015).

G. Maté et al. *The Myth of Normal: Trauma, Illness & Healing in a Toxic Culture* (London: Ebury Publishing, 2022).

M. Mischke-Reeds. *Somatic Psychotherapy Toolbox: 125 Worksheets and Exercises to Treat Trauma & Stress* (Eau Claire, WI: PESI, 2018).

M. Mischke-Reeds. *8 Keys to Practicing Mindfulness: Practical Strategies for Emotional Health and Well Being* (New York: W. W. Norton & Company, 2015).

A. Schwartz. *The Complex PTSD Treatment Manual: An Integrative, Mind-Body Approach to Trauma Recovery* (Eau Claire, WI: PESI, 2021).

A. Schwartz. *The Complex PTSD Workbook: A Mind-Body Approach to Regaining Emotional Control and Becoming Whole* (London: John Murray Press, 2020).

A. Schwartz. *The Post-Traumatic Growth Guidebook: Practical Mind-Body Tools to Heal Trauma, Foster Resilience and Awaken Your Potential* (Eau Claire, WI: PESI, 2020).

A. Schwartz. *A Practical Guide to Complex PTSD: Compassionate Strategies to Begin Healing from Childhood Trauma* (New York: Callisto Media, 2020).

A. Schwartz. *Therapeutic Yoga for Trauma Recovery: Applying the Principles of Polyvagal Theory for Self-Discovery, Embodied Healing, and Meaningful Change* (Eau Claire, WI: PESI, 2022).

A. Schwartz. *Trauma Recovery* (Louisville, CO: Sounds True, 2021).

A. Schwartz et al. *EMDR Therapy and Somatic Psychology: Interventions to Enhance Embodiment in Trauma Treatment* (New York: W. W. Norton & Company, 2018).

BA van der Kolk. *The Body Keeps the Score: Brain, Mind, and Body in the Healing of Trauma* (New York: Penguin Publishing Group, 2014).
O. Winfrey et al. *What Happened to You? Conversations on Trauma, Resilience, and Healing* (New York: Flatiron Books, 2021).

PODCASTS

Commune with Jeff Krasno. "Why Metabolic Dysfunction Kills with Dr. Sara Gottfried." September 15, 2022. https://www.youtube.com/watch?v=2o1cCDOPpWE.
Huberman Lab. "Dr. Robin Carhart-Harris: The Science of Psychedelics for Mental Health." May 22, 2023. https://hubermanlab.com/dr-robin-carhart-harris-the-science-of-psychedelics-for-mental-health/.
Huberman Lab. "Dr. Sara Gottfried: Female Hormone Optimization." January 30, 2023. https://hubermanlab.com/dr-sara-gottfried-how-to-optimize-female-hormone-health-for-vitality-and-longevity/.

PRODUCTS

- **ARTISANAL NUT CHEESE**—https://srimu.com
- **BIMUNO PREBIOTIC**—https://www.bimuno.com/
- **CURCUMIN**—https://www.thorne.com/ingredients/curcumin-phytosome?gclid=CjwKCAjwvdajBhBEEiwAeMh1U4UmrnAyPtKiZp_iWyHsef8VxJVgBphzQYebLYHyEpV_paKdKz0_vBoCfEYQAvD_BwE
- **HANU**—https://www.hanuhealth.com/
- **LEVELS**—https://www.levelshealth.com/
- **ONEGEVITY BY THORNE**—https://www.thorne.com/onegevity-health-intelligence
- **OURA RING**—https://ouraring.com
- **PROLON**—https://prolonfast.com/
- **PURELEAN FIBER**—https://www.pureencapsulationspro.com/purelean-sup-reg-sup-fiber-improved.html
- **THORNE FIBERMEND**—https://www.thorne.com/products
- **VIOME**—https://www.viome.com/
- **WHOOP**—https://www.whoop.com

TREATMENTS/ORGANIZATIONS/PROGRAMS/WEBSITES

- **ALCOHOLICS ANONYMOUS**—https://www.aa.org/
- **BLUE WAVE MEDICINE**—https://www.bluewavemedicine.com
- **BRAINSPOTTING**—https://brainspotting.com
- **ELENA BROWER**—https://elenabrower.com/

- **EYE MOVEMENT DESENSITIZATION AND REPROCESSING (EMDR)**—https://www.emdr.com/what-is-emdr/
- **FUNCTIONAL NUTRITION ALLIANCE**—https://www.fxnutrition.com
- **HAKOMI INSTITUTE**—https://hakomiinstitute.com/
- **THE INSTITUTE FOR FUNCTIONAL MEDICINE**—https://www.ifm.org/
- **KRIPALU CENTER FOR YOGA & HEALTH**—https://kripalu.org/
- **MARCUS INSTITUTE OF INTEGRATIVE HEALTH**—https://www.jeffersonhealth.org/clinical-specialties/integrative-medicine
- **MANUELA MISCHKE-REEDS**—https://manuelamischkereeds.com/books/
- **MULTIDISCIPLINARY ASSOCIATION FOR PSYCHEDELIC STUDIES**—https://maps.org/
- **ANDREA NAKAYAMA**—https://www.andreanakayama.com/
- **PALOUSE MINDFULNESS**—an online mindfulness-based stress reduction course that is free at https://palousemindfulness.com
- **STEPHEN W. PORGES, PHD**—https://www.stephenporges.com/
- **SAN FRANCISCO ZEN CENTER**—https://www.sfzc.org/locations/tassajara
- **DR. ARIELLE SCHWARTZ**—https://drarielleschwartz.com/
- **SIANNA SHERMAN**—https://www.siannasherman.com/
- **SOMATIC EXPERIENCING INTERNATIONAL**—https://traumahealing.org

INDEX